Here For Now

Living Well with Cancer
Through Mindfulness

Here For Now

Living Well with Cancer Through Mindfulness

Second Edition

Elana Rosenbaum, MS, LICSW

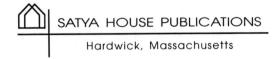
SATYA HOUSE PUBLICATIONS
Hardwick, Massachusetts

Published in the United States of America
by Satya House Publications
Post Office Box 122
Hardwick, Massachusetts 01037-0122
www.satyahouse.com

Manufactured in the United States of America.

Second Edition

ISBN 978-0-9729191-2-8

The meditation on page 25 first appeared in *Tricycle,* Spring 2005.

Cover and book design by Julie Murkette
Author photo by Stephen DiRado

This book is dedicated to my husband David,
who held my hand and comforted me with his presence
when I was ill and keeps my spirit alive and joyous
through all my days.

IN APPRECIATION

To all who pray for me, love me, and sustain me, thank you.
I am filled with gratitude.

In appreciation,
May these blessings be received:

*May the one who was a source of blessing for our ancestors bring the
blessings of healing upon those who we name in our hearts —
a healing of body and a healing of spirit.
May those in whose care they are entrusted be gifted with wisdom
and skill in their care.
May family and friends who surround them be gifted with love and
openness, strength and trust in their care.
May we all be blessed.
May we all be well.
May we all live in love and freedom.*

TABLE OF CONTENTS

FOREWORD

There was a moment standing at the foot of Elana's bed in the Bone Marrow Transplant Unit gazing down on her bald head and feeling the labored breathing of the pneumonia she had contracted after her stem cell treatment, when I thought we might actually lose her that very day. Apparently a lot of other people, including some of the staff on the Unit, thought so too. But Elana did not die. She came back from what looked, from the outside, to be death's very door. Her life force just hung on, against all odds, and she somehow hung in with it.

It didn't surprise those of us who knew her . . . Elana Rosenbaum "defines" commitment, resolve, determination, and stubborn perseverance. In my experience of it, having worked closely together in the Stress Reduction Clinic and the Center for Mindfulness at the UMass Medical Center for close to twenty years, that is how she approaches everything; her work, her meditation practice, her life. What it feels like ultimately, radiating out of her and all around her, is love. You can feel it in these pages, in which she shares with us her wild ride, and even more importantly, her dharma energies and wisdom. One testament to her energies and wisdom is that, in the months following her discharge from the Transplant Unit, a good number of the staff signed up to take the Stress Reduction Program, having witnessed something in her that comes in large measure out of her meditation practice, and wanting to acquire it for themselves and perhaps as an aid for other patients facing the same rock wall of being brought to death's door in order to save them.

Elana embodies in herself everything she teaches others, for the most part now cancer patients. Her authority, her authenticity, and her personal commitment entrain just about everyone into the beauty already to be found in their own lives, often obscured by the shadow of their disease, and all the ghosts of fear and pain and turmoil associated with it.

You have to know Elana to really appreciate her luminosity, her effervescence, and her unbridled enthusiasm for life. She radiates the determination and, strange to say, the innocence and purity of the *Little Engine That Could* like nobody else I have ever met. Now, in these pages, you have a priceless opportunity to get to know her and share in her remarkable energies. You have here the priceless opportunity to explore the power of mindfulness in the service of coming to terms with things as they actually are — a good way to think of healing — and above all, you have the priceless opportunity to come to know yourself, intimately, in ways that may make all the difference. As the poet, Kabir, put it, "Fantastic! Don't let a chance like this go by!"

Jon Kabat-Zinn

PREFACE TO THE SECOND EDITION

Sometimes people ask me, "Are you cured?"

"Cured of what?" I ask them.

I know they are referring to cancer, which in my case is lymphoma, but cancer has never been the problem. It is my attitude towards cancer, not whether it recurs, that is relevant.

Of course, I like it when my energy is good and my body is functioning smoothly. I still get nervous before CT Scans. But this passes. I continue to learn that I don't have to like what happens and that feelings — be they pleasant, unpleasant, or neutral — are transitory. When I don't cling to what I wish was present, but instead keep myself open to what is occurring, there is no problem. Practicing being mindful of my attitude and my actions makes a difference.

So, I thank people for caring, tell them, "I am well," and we move on. My preference is to talk about freedom and happiness. I am interested personally and professionally in how it can be achieved and maintained.

Mindfulness remains central to my life. I bring it into my practice as a psychotherapist and teach it in the workshops I lead. I'm now also teaching medical school students and find myself emphasizing the importance of kindness and compassion, as well as ethical behavior. There seems to be a new hunger to apply mindfulness to medicine, a practice that is being increasingly used and researched.

I feel honored that my own experience has inspired a large research study that is currently measuring the effectiveness of mindfulness for patients who are undergoing stem cell transplants. I am the consultant to this study. I also continue to teach meditation in different venues and to study it myself.

So, it is with much gratitude that I introduce this second edition of *Here for Now*.

I am alive. I am well. I continue to challenge myself to be fully here for now.

What about you?

Elana Rosenbaum
January 10, 2007

ACKNOWLEDGMENTS

This book could not have come into being without the help of many people who consistently supported me with their unflagging generosity of spirit, love, kindness and care. Without them I would not be alive today. I'd like to thank my husband David Levitin for his patience and dedication in caring for me and reading and re-reading my manuscript and checking it for grammatical errors even at the end of a long work day; my brother Bob Rosenbaum who took time off from work and humored me and rearranged all the spices in my cabinet when I could barely eat; my niece Bekka who visited me in the hospital and cheered me up with ice cream cone tattoos to paste on my bald head; my niece Anna who is lovely inside and out; my cousins, especially Walter, Jon, Sherry and Jane Sass, Susan Giordano, and Christine Sass, my sisters-in-law Judi Davis and Pat Levitin and my brother-in-law Peter Levitin and his family: Jennifer, Gregory, Cynthia, and Stephen.

I also thank my dharma brothers and sisters who are my colleagues at The Center for Mindfulness and give me spiritual and emotional sustenance. I give thanks to Jon Kabat-Zinn for hiring me as a teacher in the Stress Reduction Program all those many years ago and having faith in me even when I doubted myself. Jon, you have changed my life; your love, generosity, and vision continue to inspire me. Saki Santorelli, who now directs the Center, has been a special friend and brother, fighting me, supporting me and loving me. Thank you for your wisdom, love and poetic soul. My dear, dear friends and soul sisters, Florence Meyer and Melissa Blacker, who carry on the tradition and enhance it by their shining wisdom and beauty; my roommate and fellow traveler Ferris Urbanowski, with whom I've shared many adventures; my fellow teachers, Fernando de Torrijos, Pam Erdman, James Carmody, Diana Kamila, Nerina Hendry, Ellen Wingard, Rafaela Morales, and Debby Beck. Also Larry Horowitz, and his wife Karen, whose photo of women supporting each other during a birthing still hangs in my house; Ann Skillings, Leigh Emery, Michael and Rachel Bratt, Judy and Ira Ockene, Jean Baril, Leslie Lynch, Carol Lewis, Roberta Lewis, Betty Flodin, Diane Spinney and all others who have entered the doors of the Stress Reduction Clinic be they staff, patients or interns.

I feel very blessed to have the benefit of wonderful teachers, Larry Rosenberg, my first meditation teacher, Sharon Salzberg, Kamala Masters, Joseph Goldstein, Sylvia Boorstein, Steve Armstrong, Corrado Pensa, Franz Moeckl, and others at the Insight Meditation Society in Barre, Massachusetts, my home away from home, where I replenished and found a new balance. Thank you for all that Metta. I always felt bathed in your love and wisdom.

May everyone have friends as wonderful as Susan Rashba, Susan Bauer-Wu, Paula Solomon, Suzanne Hanser, Christine Nevins, Penina Adelman, Evelyn Harris, Emily and Jeff Bright, Stephanie Colson-Stuhr, Myra Graubard, Betsy Wertheimer, Sheila Trugman and Dick Rudnick, Dr. Dale Magee and Melanie, Pam Powel, Phyllis Pilgrim, Ann and Bob Perschel, Gayle Golden, Myron and Suri Maron, Leslie Bourne, Ann Massion, Ruth Westheimer, and Rabbi Jay Rosenbaum.

I thank my support group of fabulous strong, smart women and fellow survivors, my Stem Cell Sisters, Linda Pape, Agnetha Brown, Janet Birbara, and Peggy Steinberg.

I also want to thank my Shabat Meditation Group who meditated and prayed with me and for me, especially Alan Shapiro, Ira Grotick, Eddie Hauben, Jan Hauben and Bob Hiller.

My medical care has been exceptional. I'd like to thank the entire medical staff of the bone marrow transplant unit at the University of Massachusetts Medical Center in 1996, in particular my oncologist Dr. Pam Becker, who always took the time to explain everything to me carefully and completely so I could understand it, Dr. Peter

Quesenberry, who was on call and knew what to do when my condition was critical, my extraordinary nurses, Heidi Waitkus, Diane Sawyer, Ann McDougle and the staff in the infusion room and blood donor center, Bill Levy, my nurse practitioner, and Cathy Butler. I'd also like to thank Dr. Karen Ballen, Dr. Chris Seidler and Dr. Arnie Friedman for being caring and smart oncologists who know how to treat the whole person.

I'd like to thank my psychotherapist, Dr. Roberta Apfel for being the good parent every one wishes to have. Your wisdom, guidance and support provided fertile soil for me to take root and grow strong. I also want to thank my personal trainer, Cheryl Mita, whose unflagging patience and expertise helped me build up my muscles and keeps me fit after the assault of chemotherapy.

This book would not have come into being without the encouragement and talent of my writing coach and editor Laura Porter, or Julie Murkette who's done a mammoth and impressive job of supporting me and this project. She edited and formatted the text, created the cover design and helped me birth this book. Thank you.

I also feel very grateful to the many other people who sent me cards, well wishes and love along the way. Please know that I appreciate all your care and thoughtfulness.

May we all be well.

INTRODUCTION

"The present moment is a precious moment." I say this over and over to the patients I see as a psychotherapist and in the mindfulness-based stress reduction classes I've been teaching for the last twenty years. I also repeat it to myself. It's a reminder, a wake-up call to pay attention and be present, here, now, in this moment, with *whatever* is happening, without judgment. This helps me stay current and not get lost in what is beyond my ability to change.

Reminding myself to stay awake and be present has been a guiding principle in my life, at work, and at home, through happy times and sad. I've been lucky. This practice of meditation has been part of my life for almost thirty years and I've had the good fortune to use it as part of my work since 1984. At that time I began teaching in the Mindfulness-based Stress Reduction Program, which was the first mind/body program in the nation, founded by Jon Kabat-Zinn at the University of Massachusetts Medical Center in 1979. Over 16,000 people have gone through this program and been helped in coping with emotional and physical disorders such as anxiety, headaches, cancer, AIDS, heart disease, gastro-intestinal disorders, psoriasis, fibromyalgia, pain, and stress-related symptoms. In the spring of 1995, when I was diagnosed with Non-Hodgkin's lymphoma, I became one of them. Staying present and paying attention *without judgment* was vital if I didn't want to get lost and swallowed up by self-pity or despair. It became imperative that I focus on what I did have control over-my attitude-in order to maintain a sense of well-being.

"There's more right with you than wrong," I'd tell my classes, "even in the face of a life-threatening illness." But acting on this belief and staying happy requires effort. My diagnosis forced me to confront habits that kept me from being well. It forced me to pay attention and really notice what helped me stay well and what I needed to let go or change. Caring for myself properly meant I *really had to listen to my body and nurture myself, mind and body.* I needed to remind myself to come back to this moment again and again. I needed to maintain an open, steady heart and forgive myself if I strayed. I also needed to be able to accept support. My intention and commitment NOT to SUFFER became paramount in my ability to cope with the rapidity of change that the diagnosis of cancer wrought in my life.

"May I be safe and protected. May I be happy. May I be healthy. May I live with ease." These are words of a loving-kindness meditation that I learned from Sharon Salzberg at the Insight Meditation Society where I went for meditation retreats. I'd repeat these words to myself as I'd walk along, as I sat in waiting rooms, as I lay in bed receiving chemotherapy and throughout my daily activities. When I noticed my mind drifting I'd wake myself up by focusing on a sound in the room or by noticing the in and out movement of breath in my body. I used my meditation practice to help me connect to the sources of strength and support within and around me.

Here for Now began its life as a journal when I was first diagnosed. It included poems, illustrations and doodles that arose spontaneously as I worked to maintain my equanimity. I wrote to sort out my feelings and restore a sense of calm and quiet to the home inside of me. Sometimes the pictures reflected silent screams of anguish or wild lows of frustration so deeply embedded in mind and body that only color and form could represent them. Writing and drawing allowed my internal states to come out and be released. As I recovered, I continued to keep a record of my struggles to maintain a sense of perspective and balance. I wanted to use my experience and learn from it. I hoped to be able to use it to help others if they too became ill or challenged in maintaining a sense of health and wellness.

I was determined not to suffer. I did my best not to resist how I felt, even in the face of frequent tests and procedures, chemotherapy and a subsequent stem cell transplant. Yet when I felt most depleted and at greatest risk I also felt most complete, suffused with love, peace and calm. Only as I began to become stronger and able to do more did I become less content, my wanting mind restless and impatient with the slowness of my recovery. Now that I had survived it seemed that my challenge to stay well and be happy was harder than ever.

I love the phrase from the I Ching that says perseverance furthers, but during the period of my recovery I often identified with the runners in the Boston marathon right after Heartbreak Hill. I used to watch the marathon with my sister-in-law, Judi. Our position was beyond Heartbreak Hill but still miles before the finish line. As Anna, my niece, less than a year old, slept contentedly beside us in her baby carriage, Judi and I stood in the cold, bundled up, clapping and shouting to encourage the runners on. It was obvious that many were tired but they kept on, some limping, some walking, others going at a steady pace, powered by training, will, effort and their dream of completing this famous race. We supported them, yelling at the top of our lungs as they approached, "You can do it, Go! Only a little more. Go! You can make it."

As I kept on doing my best to keep my spirits up through a series of blood transfusions, anemia, and isolation following my transplant, I was forced to confront physical limitations. It became clear that the more I could let go and accept these limitations the better I felt and the freer I became. The more I lived in the present moment as it was, rather than what I wished it would be, the happier I felt.

In my MBSR classes I emphasized the importance of living fully, no matter what is happening, and the need to put oneself into whatever one is doing all the way. My models were *The Little Engine that Could* and Dr. Seuss's characters in *Oh, The Places You'll Go.* Seuss says, "Step with care and great tact and remember that Life's a Great Balancing Act."

Nothing stays the same, why should I? When I did return to work I no longer felt like the person I had known for over fifty years, the me that could take life for granted. This caused its own stress. I wanted every moment to be important and precious but I couldn't sustain the attentional focus that I was demanding of myself. I forgot that every moment is precious, regardless of what it holds and that it would take some time and flexibility to re-assess my priorities and find a new balance.

It's now been nine years since my transplant. My brother and his family have moved away, but I still go to the Boston marathon. Now as I stand there I find myself with tears in my eyes. I identify with the runners. As they pass I appreciate their attitude and spirit. I see how hard they are working. I know the importance of intention, dedication, practice, and putting your whole self into whatever you choose to do. Now when I work with cancer patients, newly diagnosed and fearful about the outcome of chemotherapy, I am their coach, rooting for them and their endurance of spirit and hope.

You can do it. Yes, you can.

As I am allowed to age and be here, gratitude fills me. When I lead a retreat or work with cancer patients teaching them meditation, whether I am sitting with them in my office or on the transplant unit at the Dana Farber Cancer Institute or at the University of Massachusetts Medical School, I still quote the gatta, a poem, by Thich Nhat Hahn:

> *Breathing in I calm,*
> *Breathing out I smile.*
> *Dwelling in the Present Moment*
> *It is a precious moment.*

We are here and alive now. Rest in the moment and be free of sorrow. We can be happy and live with safety, ease and well-being. This moment we have choices. Next moment, who knows?

Here for Now is about living well and facing life's challenges with strength, and grace, an open heart, a clear mind and a steadiness of purpose. The guided meditations and exercises come directly from my own experience. You may use them at any time, and in any order.

We are all unique and wonderful. In facing ourselves with compassion and opening to what is true, we become free. My goal in writing this book and sharing my journey is to facilitate a fullness of being that says, "Yes" to love and grief, happiness and sorrow, adventure and tedium, "Yes" to mistakes, and "Yes," to continued learning. Living in this way requires commitment, hard work, and effort . . . and faith in the possibility of happiness and freedom now.

HOW TO USE THIS BOOK

Here for Now combines narrative with meditations and exercises. The story is written in chronological order and can be read straight through. While reading you may pause at any time and bring awareness to any thoughts, sensations or feelings that are evoked. Feel free to doodle, jot down reflections or stop and become aware of your breath. The meditations and exercises can be done at any time, either after each chapter or later. You can use them repeatedly. You may want to experiment, experiencing each one for a period of time before you settle on one to use on a regular basis. Choose what resonates with you best. Remember to be patient and kind to yourself allowing the moment to unfold without striving to make something happen. Be as free of expectations as possible so you can explore and discover each moment anew, witnessing what arises without judgment.

It is recommended that all meditations be done in a quiet and protected environment where you practice for a set period of time without interruption. These meditations are also available on a CD that can be ordered or you can have someone read them to you or record them yourself to guide you until you are familiar with them. The more you use the meditations the greater benefit you will receive. Trust your own inner wisdom and let it be your guide. Your intention and commitment to this process is more important than achieving a particular state.

The Consent Form

Before people were allowed to participate in the Stress Reduction Program they had to commit themselves to participating fully in the program which meant attending a weekly two-and-a half hour session that met for eight weeks as well as an all day session held on a weekend after the sixth class. They also needed to agree to do their homework which consisted of a forty-five minute daily meditation alternating between a body scan meditation, yoga, or awareness of breathing. If they said, "Yes, I'm willing to do this," they then signed a consent form that said ". . . .the risks, benefits and possible side effects of the program have been explained to me fully."

As I'd hand out the form I'd think, "Risks? What risks? You're being offered an opportunity to practice meditation. You have eight weeks of support and help in being with yourself and taking time to nurture yourself. You'll be in a community of like-minded people all of whom are dedicated to being well. You go at your own pace. You are responsible for yourself. The yoga we do is a series of very gentle stretches. You can be as verbally participatory as you are comfortable being. There's nothing you have to do except take the time to stop and inquire, with awareness and kindness, into the present moment."

Here's what I've discovered about them:

Risks

- You can get to know yourself better; insight can come without warning
- You might experience feelings of joy
- You might experience feelings of pain
- You might notice ways in which you are not balanced
- Change. You could change
- Change requires adjustments to regain a sense of balance
- Old memories could return
- You'll probably have to readjust your schedule to do the homework

- You'll have to let some things go
- Relationships might be experienced differently both with yourself and others
- You'll be facing the unknown-yourself
- You might not like what you discover
- You will be challenged
- Challenge requires effort
- You will have to take responsibility for yourself and your actions

BENEFITS

- Less mental anguish
- A greater sense of well-being
- Freedom
- Happiness, joy, peace
- A greater sense of balance in your life
- Mindfulness: Clear seeing and understanding
- A quieter mind
- A sense of wholeness, vastness, space, connection
- Wisdom

POSSIBLE SIDE EFFECTS

- New understanding
- A more expansive perspective
- Wonder fullness

Life is filled with risks, benefits and side effects. I've signed the consent form. How about you?

EXERCISE: THE CONSENT FORM

My Intention/Goals are:

1.

2.

3.

Now, ask yourself if you are willing to make a commitment to yourself to work towards your goals mindfully with love and compassion. If the answer is "yes" you may sign below.

Your intention to be well, and pay attention mindfully to whatever arises with love and care will powerfully affect the outcome of your goals.

I, _____

commit myself to actively engage in the practice of mindfulness for

_____ and work toward

(Fill in length of time you are willing to give it a chance.)

my goals to the best of my efforts.

Signed _____

A GUIDED MEDITATION

TO BEGIN, ASSUME A POSITION that supports your ability to be awake and alert as well as comfortable. Gently close your eyes and bring awareness to sound. Let yourself receive what you are hearing, and notice what comes without striving to make something happen. You may hear sounds in the room or sounds outside the room, or no sounds at all. Simply listen and notice how the sounds you hear change from moment to moment.

When you feel ready you can let your attention shift to your breathing. If you like, you can put your hands on your belly and feel it as it rises with the in-breath and falls with the out-breath. Really feel each breath as it enters and leaves the body. Notice its rhythm and explore its length and depth, observing how it changes in response to a thought or feeling. Notice the way you are breathing, through your mouth or the nose, or maybe a little of both. There may be a tendency to want to change how you are breathing, but we are practicing allowing ourselves to accept whatever is happening and noticing that moment by moment things change. The breath changes and you change. Nothing stays the same, yet there is constancy. The breath reminds us that we are here and alive: let it be your anchor to the present moment.

If you like, as you breathe in, knowing you're breathing in, you can imagine that you're breathing in health and vitality. On the out breath, knowing you're breathing out, you can imagine you're releasing toxins, along with any worries or fears that you'd like to let go. Notice all you can about the breath, staying with it as it comes in and as it goes out.

If physical sensations are strong, they will capture your attention; and you can breathe with them, sending care and compassion to the sensation as you notice it. Inhale, breathing in oxygen and nutrients and sending them to any part of the body that needs them, especially to any areas that are particularly sensitive. Breathe out, releasing any tension or tightness that you may notice. Breathe with the sensation, softening into it and noticing how it changes, calming yourself as you enter into it with your breath.

Observe what arises, with kindness, without judging any reactions you may be experiencing and letting each moment be a new one to enter afresh.

If you become aware that you are thinking, you can label it, "thought" and gently but firmly return your attention to the breath. It is normal for your mind to wander. Simply notice what captures your attention and bring it back. If it's helpful you can imagine that you're in a glass-bottom boat, observing fish as they swim through the water, or observing clouds moving through a vast sky on a clear day.

Be in harmony with each breath, each moment, and know that in giving yourself this time to develop awareness and a steadiness of attention you are nourishing spirit, head and heart. Let it be an adventure, and in the silence and the stillness that comes with practice you'll discover wonders here for you, now.

SECTION I

THE TREASURE

Sometimes we have to travel far to discover what is near.

There is a wonderful children's book, *The Treasure* by Uri Shulevitz. In it, a very poor man named Isaac dreams of finding a treasure in a city very far from his home. Isaac tries ignoring his dream but it won't go away. So one day he packs his things, puts on a heavy coat and hat, and sets off. He travels over hills and dales, fields and mountains. It is a long hard journey but he perseveres. Sometimes people stop and help him but often he goes alone. When he reaches his destination he discovers a guard standing at the very spot where the treasure is supposed to be. Day after day Isaac returns to this spot but each time he finds the guard stationed there. After many days, the guard, not understanding why Isaac returns to this spot, turns to him and asks, "Old man, why are you here?" Learning about his dream, the guard laughs.

"Foolish man," he says, "if I believed in dreams I'd go to the town where a man named Isaac lives and I'd go to his house and dig under his stove. A treasure is buried there."

Isaac thanks the guard and sets off again for the long journey home. When he arrives, he does as the guard instructed and discovers jewels and gold. In appreciation to the guard he sends him some jewels. He also builds a chapel for travelers with a sign that says, *"Sometimes we have to travel far to discover what is near."*

I first heard this story from my friend and colleague, Florence Meyer, who told it to her stress reduction class. Observing the class, I was captivated as she described how Isaac "kicked open his door." To demonstrate this, Florence took a breath and thrust out her own leg, giving us a sense of the energy and force Isaac needed to venture out into the unknown in search of a treasure he had seen only in a dream. As she told the story, I found my eyes tearing up. The story seemed to symbolize the distance I had traveled to discover the treasure buried inside of me.

To come home to myself and find that I am a treasure feels like a miracle. It's sweet and simple and seems to happen each time I can let go of my harsh internal monitor or my expectations of how I THINK things should be. If I can steady myself and simply investigate the sensation in my body or the thought that's causing me to be angry or hurt or disappointed *without judgment*, a deep letting go, a melting of old defenses and hurts comes. I can truly be at home, at peace, quiet and still joy bubbles up and I'm lighter and freer.

Buddhism talks about suffering and the end of suffering. "Cling to nothing," the texts say. "Everything is impermanent." My mind knows this but I don't like it. Letting go doesn't come easy for me. When I quiet down, rather than instant happiness I sometimes feel a lingering sadness, a heaviness located in the center of my chest in the area of the heart. Feeling this isn't pleasant.

"Sometimes it takes a while for grief to leave the body," Sylvia Boorstein, a teacher of mine, reassured me on a retreat. Sylvia's statement comforted me. She spoke to me with sympathy and understanding. There was no blaming or judging. She didn't correct me or make me feel like a failure as a meditator. Her response helped me let go of my unhappiness at not being happy. Perhaps, I thought, I just needed more time to release old patterns and hurts, imagined and real, from my past. I needed to trust that this moment, here for me now, was the treasure, and there was NOTHING I had to do but allow it to unfold. It helped to take the time to be on retreat, another treasure, surrounded by good people, great food, and a lovely setting. The only demand on me was that I be considerate of others and not come into the meditation hall late, be noisy or push ahead in the food line. I could do that.

Cancer motivated me to use the time I had as fully as possible. It pushed me to examine what *really* made me happy and what *really* allowed me to be well. Until I confronted death and the mini deaths of hair loss, identity changes, physical and mental limitations, I could be lazy. I didn't really have to let go, pay attention and be present. Chemotherapy did more than eradicate cancer cells. It also seemed to burn away some of the neurotic underpinnings of my life, the if only's. If only I were taller than five feet. If only my memory were better. If only I was smarter, wiser, thinner, more patient. My effort to be well absorbed my attention. I couldn't afford to be angry or overly self-critical: it zapped too much energy. I needed to focus on what could support and enliven me: the resources and riches buried under my stove in my very own house.

Like Isaac, I am not young, beautiful or rich. I'm ethnic-looking and I sweat. I can be schmaltzy and very emotional. I'm stubborn, impractical and determined. I also persevere in the face of challenges and am willing to take risks.

I was born in 1943 to Jewish parents in Mt. Vernon, New York. My father, "smilin' Jack" Rosenbaum, was the older of two sons. He was a paint salesman, charming, warm and impractical. He used to remind me to smile, which I didn't appreciate at the time. My mother would have to urge him to get to work in the morning. Dad preferred sitting at his desk, going through papers and jotting down inspirational sayings from books he got in the library. Later, when I'd ride with him in his car, which also served as his office as he drove through the south Bronx going from paint store to paint store, I'd notice some of these sayings in different colored inks on a sticker on the dashboard:

> *You cannot prevent the birds of sorrow*
> *from flying over your head,*
> *But you can prevent them*
> *from building nests in your hair.*

"Jaack! It's late!" My mother, a 4'11" dynamo with big breasts that she always complained about, would yell at my father as he sat at his desk writing down yet another saying. Dad had no sense of time. He was very thoughtful and went out of his way to please my mother but he wanted to do it his way and in his own time frame.

"Who wears the pants?" he'd cry out when he thought she was pushing him around too much. Mom, who worried more than Dad and was less easily satisfied, could get VERY angry and frustrated at him. Growing up poor, the second youngest of eight children, she worried about money. Conscious of being a child of poor immigrants in upstate New York, she felt the effects of anti-Semitism and felt different. Born between a sickly older sister, Ethel, and a boy, Larry, who as a boy and the youngest was special, she felt inadequate and unloved. Mom, warm, intuitive and loving, also wished she were richer, didn't live with her in-laws and had gone to college. She was very sensitive and easily hurt. I, her daughter, the oldest, also struggled with feeling I wasn't good enough and couldn't satisfy her no matter how hard I tried. I did not think I was a treasure . . . but I wanted to be one, as did she. Neither of us believed it was possible.

When I was in my thirties and divorced, I decided it was time to stop complaining and give myself what I felt had been denied me growing up. I gave myself ballet lessons, I began playing the saxophone in a sax choir for adult beginners, and I painted a mural on the walls in my bedroom that covered the entire room. I'd change it as the mood took me. Across from my bed were birches, graceful and aesthetic. Leaves grew lushly on each branch in different shades of green. The sky was blue and cloudless. It was springtime and serenity greeted me as I woke up. On the large wall to the right of my bed was a very large oak with broad branches supporting creatures of the imagination.

I spent days and nights painting the trunk, branches, and roots of the tree. I used house paint, pastels and acrylics. My father had given me colored tints and I mixed my own paint. The wall was large and I used it all, painting my emotions, my passion, my fears and uncertainties. Coming home late at night, taking out my brushes, the different mediums I used for color and texture, I filled every part of the wall and moved to the door and over the entranceway. My tree was broad and full. Its roots were equally large and wide, filling a greater part of the bottom of the wall. The tree had depth, variety, and color. I'd add to it late at night, creating new images or adding more color to its branches. It appeared strong and solid and graceful. It reached out and up.

When my mother came to visit me she looked at the mural, sighed and said, "I guess that's you."

My name is Elana. It means tree in Hebrew. Elana, tree, Elan, spirit. Elana, the name I had been called when I spent a year in Israel when I was a junior in college. Elana, a name with a lovely cadence, promise, possibilities, connecting me to historic roots and offering me a future of hope and freedom. I was not born with this name. I gave it to myself after my divorce in 1975, when I returned to my maiden name, Rosenbaum. I no longer felt like Ellen Rosenbaum, that girl from Mt. Vernon who was so insecure and inadequate, so unhappy.

During my illness, as I struggled to find the treasure of equanimity, the image of a tree came back to me. This time I focused not on its trunk or branches, but on its roots, imagining them going deep, deep down, pushing through crumbling soil and moving towards moisture and nourishment. The roots support the tree. They are its foundation, allowing it to rise high and put out branches and leaves that touch the sun, the air, the wind, and the rain.

Each time I return to my breath, each time I come back to the present moment, I imagine my roots becoming stronger, keeping me upright as I move through seasons and climate change, braving the elements of my mind, my wants and desires, disappointments and losses, to bring me home again, to the treasures that are here now.

THE TREASURE: A GUIDED MEDITATION

The Treasure is a very old story. It reminds us that one may not need to spend years seeking outside of ourselves and traveling long distances to find happiness and fulfillment when the treasure lies within, at home all the time. This meditation and the meditations that follow are designed to help us return home to ourselves. The attitude that you bring to them is as important as the meditation itself. See if you can treat them as a time for self-nurturing and support. Let them be a gift to yourself, a voyage without any expectations. It's important not to strive for something to happen. Simply notice what arises as an explorer might, with a sense of adventure and curiosity. If you notice any judging thoughts do your best to let go of them and simply return to the present moment. Your commitment and intention to be more aware and free is important.

Carefully choose the time and place you do this meditation. Let it be a sanctuary, protected in time and space, a treasure in itself, where you can relax and still your mind. Select a time when you will be free of interruptions or any obligations except to yourself. You may read this meditation slowly to yourself or have a friend or partner say it to you. You may even make your own tape, with your own voice or the voice of a loved one, giving yourself permission to receive *The Treasure* now.

TO BEGIN, FIND A POSITION that is comfortable and will support your ability to relax. If you are sitting up, sit in an erect and dignified position with your chin level to the floor and your spine upright in alignment with your pelvis slightly forward, your feet touching the floor and your legs uncrossed. You can let your arms rest wherever is comfortable to you. You may also use a recliner or do this lying down, arms alongside the body and feet about six inches apart.

When you are ready, bring your attention to the treasure of breath and breathing. Bring your awareness to the sensation of inhaling and exhaling. As you breathe in, really allow yourself to feel the entire inhalation. As you breathe out, really let yourself feel the entire exhalation. You can note whether it is fast or slow, deep or shallow. Don't try to change it in any way; simply observe its rhythm.

Where are you feeling the breath? Is it at the nostrils, the chest, or in the belly? Can you follow the whole breath and feel it move the body? Do your best to follow it with as full attention as possible, letting go of everything but the sensations of breathing.

When your attention is steady on the in-breath you can say to yourself, *"I am a treasure."* On the out-breath you can say, *"May I care for and treasure my treasures."* Do this slowly and repeatedly, allowing treasures to come to you without trying to make it happen.

Notice what feelings, thoughts, or sensations arise as you repeat the phrases to yourself. Perhaps a deep gratitude and appreciation will arise as you let yourself receive the treasures already known to you and allow yourself to open to new ones. Simply notice what arises, observing without judging. If you find your mind wandering, gently but firmly bring it back to the next breath, and the phrases, the treasure of this practice, and your ability to breathe and be here now.

Saying the phrases to yourself, with each breath, freely acknowledge some treasures you already know you have. You can name positive characteristics and gifts that you've been given, such as the treasure of being kind-hearted, caring, funny, curious, wise, or patient. Give yourself permission to name and appreciate these characteristics. They are valuable resources and gifts. If negativity arises, breathe it out and let it go and return to the phrase, *"I am a treasure. May I treasure my treasures."*

You can use this time to acknowledge the treasure of having loved ones and of loving and being loved. Let these people enter your awareness and give thanks to them for being in your life.

You can allow yourself to name your treasures, again and again, saying them to yourself, experiencing and receiving them, as you continue following the movement of your breath and repeating to yourself, *"I am a treasure . . . I am blessed with treasures, treasures within and treasures without. May I use my gifts wisely, May I acknowledge my treasures, May I give as well as receive."* Use phrases that resonate with you and name as many treasures as come to mind.

If treasures are not noted, that is fine too; you can treasure the moment and your being present to it. Treasures may come to you that surprise you. Perhaps you'll notice the sounds around you, the ordinary sounds of life coming and going and treasure being able to hear and receive them.

Notice your belly as it continues to move, rising on the in-breath and descending on the out-breath, flowing like the tides of the sea, coming and going. If you like, you can imagine the breath smoothing what it touches, washing away debris and then returning again with fresh air. Be aware of the natural rhythm of your breath as it revitalizes mind and body by cleansing and renewing breath by breath. Let yourself follow the treasure of breath which brings you home, connecting you to life itself, the mystery and the treasure.

Breathing in and out you can always return to your breath, to the present moment letting it calm and quiet you. You can let yourself be rocked by breath, like a baby by its parent. And the breath will continue flowing . . . as you wake up to who you are, your beauty and goodness . . . your treasures, here for you now.

May you treasure your treasures.

Exercise: My Treasures

IF YOU LIKE, YOU CAN jot down a list of your treasures to remind yourself that they are present and reside with you wherever you are and whatever you are doing. You may also find photographs of treasures and make a collage or choose to draw or represent a treasure. It can be an object of nature, person, place, or symbol. If you choose to draw let color and form appear without straining to make something happen. Remember, this exercise is for you; whatever emerges is fine. Enjoy.

MEDITATION AND THE HOKEY POKEY

You put your whole self in
You put your whole self out
You put your whole self in
And you shake it all about
You do the Hokey Pokey
And you turn yourself around
And that's what it's all about.

I have a black t-shirt that says, "Maybe the hokey-pokey is what it's all about." I love wearing it, especially when I'm teaching meditation. It seems to lighten up the room and put the intensity of mind-watching in perspective. My colleagues at the Center for Mindfulness at the University of Massachusetts Medical Center in Worcester used to laugh at me when I equated what we did to the hokey pokey. I seemed to be the only one to see the connection.

The words of the hokey pokey first came to me in the midst of a very serious ten day silent Vipassana (mindfulness) retreat. It was the late 1970's and meditation seemed a very in thing to do. I was in my 30's, single, living in Cambridge and new to meditation, coming to it out of curiosity and unhappiness. I hoped to meet people and feel more satisfied with myself and my decision to live on the East Coast. I had moved from Seattle, where I had lived for eight years, to Cambridge to be closer to my brother who lived in Boston and my parents who lived in Mt. Vernon, NY. I left an established career, good friends and a passionate but disastrous relationship. Re-establishing myself and recovering from the relationship was harder than I had anticipated. Now, a year later, I was wondering if I had made a wise choice. I thought the time and space of a retreat setting would help me lick my wounds and recover. I didn't realize that my unsettled mind would travel with me to the brown hills of northern California where I had chosen to go on retreat.

In the retreat I had nothing to do but observe myself: my ups, my downs, my likes, my dislikes. I couldn't read, talk on the telephone, or eat except at specified times. Why, I wondered, had I chosen to do this? (A familiar question.) I found it excruciating to be still and just observe the workings of my own mind. There were no distractions. I was stuck with my own discontent.

I recalled the first time I meditated. It was in Cambridge at a New Age Institute called Interface. I was one of perhaps fifteen people in a room that was small and cold. It was lined with flat mats and small cushions where people sat cross-legged facing the teacher, Larry Rosenberg. The instructions were, " Do nothing but follow the breath as it enters and leaves the body. Notice where you're feeling it most vividly and keep your attention there. If the mind wanders, simply notice it and return your attention to the breath."

Sitting upright on small round cushions in a cross-legged position on a hard floor was uncomfortable. My body ached. My mind was restless. I kept thinking, why am I doing this? Everyone else was sitting quietly and I didn't want to embarrass myself by fleeing.

I sat in a draft and wondered whether it would be OK to close the door. As I practiced focusing on my breath, noticing it as I breathed in and out, my mind didn't seem to want to cooperate. I was miserable and wanted to leave. I strained to pay attention and stay in the present moment without judging myself and felt like a failure. Meditation was supposed to calm me and help me be peaceful. Instead I seemed to either fall asleep, be irritated, restless, bored or heavy hearted. I ruminated, Should I move or keep sitting? Wanting to be a "good" meditator I didn't budge. I wanted Larry's approval and I was afraid of what he would think if I got up and closed the door. My body appeared stationary, but my mind kept going over whether to close the door or not. Rather than "let go" and stop ruminating, I kept battling myself. I felt as if I was in a torture chamber without an exit. Years later when I was teaching stress reduction I'd quote Wittgenstein who said, "The way out is through the door. Why is it that no one will take the exit?"

At the end of the weekend, Larry said, "Isn't this wonderful?" and I thought, "NO!"

Yet, I persevered. Now I had signed up for this ten day retreat and I was miserable again, caught in indecision. Should I move once more? I wished I were someplace else. Seattle? Cambridge? California? My mind wouldn't steady. Inside the gated lawn of the retreat center it was green, like New England. Beyond the gates it was brown and hilly, very Northern California, and if I kept going on one of the trails, which I did after lunch every day, I came upon a lovely and cool blue-green pond which reminded me of Seattle.

One afternoon I was doing a walking meditation, focusing my attention on lifting, moving and placing my foot on the ground, and my mind was unusually busy. As my mind pondered where to place my foot in the future I'd momentarily lose my balance. When I stumbled and noticed what my mind was doing, I'd criticize myself and then try again. This kept repeating itself over and over. Suddenly I found myself silently singing, *"You pick your right foot up, you put your right foot down. You pick your left foot up. You put your left foot down. You do the hokey pokey and you turn yourself around. That's what it's all about."*

I lightened up. I realized that I needed to turn myself around, mentally, and really commit myself to being here, where I was. I needed to connect to this earth, here. The future would take of itself. I realized that I was nowhere, only in my head. I was also resisting walking slowly. I *thought* it was boring. I was making it drudgery. I wasn't putting my whole self into it. The meditation instruction was "BE PRESENT." Where was I? Once I could acknowledge what I was *really* doing (resisting) my attitude changed. Fatigue, boredom, irritation, frustration dropped away. I was in the present moment!!! Struggle ceased. Maybe the hokey pokey is what it's all about!

The mind is so nimble it is often compared to a monkey climbing all over the place or a little puppy that needs to be trained gently but firmly to listen and be still. When I put my WHOLE self into being present with the moment I was in, it was easier to pay attention and experience the subtleties of the movements in walking. I could focus clearly on the sensation of moving my body through space — to my surprise, it was interesting. My balance also improved. I felt the support of the earth below me. I noticed my feet in contact with the ground. I felt the connection of foot to ankle, ankle to leg, and upward to the crown of my head. I felt the wonder of being able to be upright and I was all right. How wonder full.

This taste of happiness and contentment kept me meditating. Once a week I'd walk to the bookstore in Harvard Square where Larry held a meditation class. I'd go up the stairs to the room where people congregated and find a spot in a row with others in the narrow space on the floor. We'd meditate for about forty-five minutes and then Larry would give a talk, which we then discussed. After the talk I'd go out for coffee with Lewis and Herb and we'd talk some more. I had a crush on Lewis and I thought he and Herb were very funny. We laughed a lot, schmoozed and discussed LIFE. It was fun. It was stimulating. It felt meaningful. I began to feel more at home in Cambridge. My work life also improved. I got a good job as a therapist in Worcester, Massachusetts, at a large medical clinic that was also an HMO. My life was beginning to settle down.

Coincidentally, one of Larry's best friends, Jon Kabat-Zinn, was starting a Stress Reduction program in the department of medicine right down the road from where I was working. He offered free yoga classes at the hospital at lunchtime. I saw patients in the morning and did yoga at lunchtime. I'd then return to the clinic refreshed and ready to see more patients in the afternoon. Larry was going to be teaching meditation in Jon's program. He didn't have a car so I offered to drive him to the program. Every Monday for about six months I'd get up early and pick him up in Somerville. We drove the 50 minutes to Worcester, talking and talking, and laughing.

The conversation was so stimulating that I'd often miss the exit and have to go back. In the lulls of conversation we'd hear the exhaust of my little Fiat and Larry would chant "Ohm" in tune with the sound of the car. When I dropped him off he'd say, "Now I'm really going to be present today," and I'd make the same commitment. It was a challenge. Could I really listen and be with my clients that were scheduled for the day without my mind wandering?

Larry blew my image of meditation teachers as being holy and always serious. It was fun to travel with him. It was not beneath him to listen to rock and roll or comment on my love life. Once, as we were listening to the Stones singing, "You can't always get what you want . . . . you get what you need," Larry gave me a nudge. He knew I had a crush on Lewis, and Lewis liked me, but not in that way. He was trying to tell me humorously, "let go" if you want to be happy. You can't always get what you want, but you can get what you need. I didn't like this.

Larry seemed to be happy. I remember meeting him one day in Harvard Square with his friend, Corrado Pensa, a meditation teacher from Italy. I was coming home from work and feeling tired and not particularly happy, my mind focusing on what was absent in my life. Looking at Larry and Corrado made me envious; they seemed to be enjoying themselves, walking around as if they had no cares. And when I asked Larry how he was, he said, "Great."

"How are you?" he asked me.

"Not so great."

Why wasn't I happy? I asked myself. Was my unhappiness based on craving the impossible?

I kept practicing. I also entered psychotherapy.

About a year later I turned 40 and gave myself a present. I quit my job and opened my own private practice as a psychotherapist. This gave me flexible hours and more control over my time. Some things are within our control to change. Giving myself this time allowed me to be available when "Jonny," as Larry called him, had an opening for another instructor at the Stress Reduction Clinic. Now I could incorporate my training as a psychotherapist with meditation and work with people I respected. I could put my whole self into teaching: *There's more right with you than wrong. The greatest relaxation of all is to be comfortable in your own skin. The only moment we have is now.*

EXERCISE: NOTICING

STOP AND TAKE A MOMENT RIGHT NOW TO NOTICE WHAT IS IN YOUR AWARENESS.

- Are there any sounds that you are hearing right now?

- Are you aware of your body and the position it is in right now?

- Are there any particular sensations that you're feeling?

- Are you aware of your breathing?

- Can you notice what happens in the body when you breathe in?

- What about breathing out?

- Where in the body is the breath most vivid for you?

- Are you noticing any smells?

- Are there any thoughts moving through your mind?

- If you were to be asked, "How are you right now?" how would you answer that question?

AWARENESS OF BREATHING MEDITATION

It is best to do this for a set period of time,
preferably at the same time each day.

GET INTO AS COMFORTABLE a position as possible, gently close your eyes and be aware of the experience of breathing. See if you can notice the breath as it comes into and as it leaves the body. Where do you feel the breath most vividly? Is it at the nostrils, the chest, the belly? If you like, you can let your hand rest on your belly and feel it rising and falling as you breathe in and out. There's nothing you have to do. Don't try to change it or have it be any particular way. Simply notice what is happening.

You may also be aware of thoughts, of feelings, bodily sensations or sounds. Simply witness this, letting them pass without trying to change anything. If it's helpful you can imagine that you're in a glass bottom boat observing your thoughts as if they were fish swimming by or like clouds coming and going in a vast and clear sky.

When your mind wanders, gently but firmly return your attention to your breath and the motion of breathing. If you're having any particularly strong sensation or experience that captures your attention, you can bring your awareness to it and its different sensations, even breathing with it if you'd like, giving it space and holding it in awareness. When you're ready you can return to your breath as the main focus of attention. You can always open your eyes, look around, and then return to your breathing, closing your eyes again when you are ready.

You can simply tune in to your breathing any time. It can be an anchor to the present moment, a reminder that you can calm and return to a more spacious sense of being.

MINDFULNESS MEDITATION

Mindfulness Meditation is about noticing what is happening,
without judging.
SIMPLY NOTICE

It is about seeing clearly.
SIMPLY OBSERVE

It is about paying attention.
PAY ATTENTION

It is about being aware moment by moment of our experience.
BE AWARE

It is about having an open heart and mind.
HAVE AN OPEN HEART AND MIND

It is about courage and fearlessness.
WATCH WHAT ARISES

It is about impermanence.
NOTICE THAT EVERYTHING CHANGES

It is about riding the waves of our mental and physical states.
IT IS ABOUT LETTING GO

It is about giving and receiving love, compassion and wisdom.
RESTING IN THE MOMENT
PEACE ABOUNDS

THE STRESS REDUCTION CLINIC AND THE CHICKPEA

Chickpea to Cook

A chickpea leaps almost over the rim of the pot
Where it's being boiled.
    "Why are you doing this to me?"
The cook knocks him down with the ladle.
    "Don't you try to jump out.
You think I'm torturing you.
I'm giving you flavor,
So you can mix with spices and rice
And be the lovely vitality of a human being.

﷽

The Cook says,
    "I was once like you,
fresh from the ground. Then I boiled in Time,
 and boiled in the Body, two fierce boilings.
My animal-soul grew powerful.
I controlled it with practices,
And boiled some more, and boiled once beyond that,
and became your Teacher."

— Rumi, *Mathnawi*, III, 4160-4168, 4197-4208
Translated by Coleman Barks

When I first began teaching at The Stress Reduction Clinic I had no idea that the work would become so central to my life. I was impressed by the transformation I saw in the patients who attended the classes and amazed that symptom relief could occur so dramatically and in such a brief time. After having worked as a psychotherapist for lengthy periods of time, sometimes even years, observing change in a mere 8 weeks seemed like a miracle. Participants reported a higher degree of satisfaction in their quality of living and felt more optimistic about their ability to take charge of their lives. Symptom relief, as measured by a pre-class symptom checklist and post-class evaluation improved significantly. (See studies by Jon Kabat-Zinn, et.al.)

The work was satisfying, interesting and never boring. A sense of community and trust developed in the classes. Not only was it okay to be honest and talk about true feelings, fears and hopes, but actually required. I felt my soul was fed and held in a community of honest, loving, caring and courageous people, many of whom were living with very serious physical problems. I heard, "I'm not my pain," or "I'm enjoying my kids in ways I never could before," or "Maybe my problem isn't so big. My life is better than I thought."

At the same time, the pressure of being transparent, authentic and fully present while teaching was itself a cooker for my own insecurities to come to the surface. Meditation is a great purifier, but this little chickpea often felt on a high boil. My teaching was often observed by visitors, either Jon, Saki (Saki Santorelli, who now directs the program), and later, professionals who wanted to learn how we effected change and brought meditation into the mainstream. All my observers were free with suggestions and questions. "What was your intention?" they wanted to know when I asked a question, clarified a process, or stopped a person from going on and on about his or her problem. In addition, I, who struggled with the body scan and always felt very unathletic, had to develop a body awareness and learn to teach yoga. I began to see that my own internal critic was causing dis-stress. Wanting to do and say the "right thing" and give a perfect response made me self-conscious. My fear of being criticized or looking stupid caused me to lose connection to myself and to others. It created blinders that boxed me in and stopped me from helping anyone.

I'm afraid this is a common trap. It is easy to focus on the problem rather than on finding a solution to it. To demonstrate the boxes that we can create for ourselves, such as negative thinking or false perceptions, (i.e. "I'm stupid"), there is an exercise in the workbook that we have class members do during their second class. The page has nine dots on it, arranged in a square. The instructions are, "Connect the dots in four straight lines without lifting your pencil from the paper." People were often frustrated as they attempted to solve this puzzle. The solution was to go beyond the dots, and outside the box. I could show people how to move beyond the box on paper, but demonstrating how to do it in real life was harder. It meant I had to notice my own box, usually fear, self-doubt, or self-consciousness and bring attention to it, *without judgment.* Going outside the box meant *letting go* of my fear and reconnecting to my direct experience of the moment.

Once, a member of the class described a flashback she had during her body scan meditation, a 45-minute meditation bringing awareness into the body, part by part, breath by breath. Her description of her trauma grew more and more vivid and I could see and feel the members of the class becoming more and more uncomfortable. The waves of emotion rose higher and higher with each sentence she spoke. Every time I tried to bring her back to the present moment, she ignored me and continued on. I felt stuck. All of us were experiencing the trauma along with her. I couldn't seem to stop it.

"Oh," I thought, "I'm really cooked now. I'm losing the whole class." It made me even more uncomfortable that I was being observed by a visiting meditation teacher, a good friend of Jon's and highly respected.

Finally, I forced myself to stop thinking and trying so hard to stop her from re-experiencing her trauma. I said to her and the class, "I don't know what to do. I don't know how I can help you." Silence. Pause. I had everyone's attention. People were upright in their chairs, wide awake and on alert, waiting to see what would happen next and then, the woman who had been caught in the violence of her past began crying, and she was present again as I held her hand and we all breathed a sigh of relief. She was back in the class with us. We could relax again.

Letting go is as easy as an out-breath. It seems as if it should be simple to return to something observable and concrete in the present, but it actually requires a lot of effort and is humbling. How sweet it feels to bring attention to my breath and let go of judgment. Yet, doing so means I have to stay on alert and make the conscious effort to notice when I am lost in judgment or negativity. It took time and practice for me to stop questioning whether I was good enough to be teaching meditation. It was a relief to realize that I didn't need to know the answer to every question; that it was fine to take the time to consider a response rather than react quickly out of anxiety.

Observing transformation in the patients inspired me. I remember a man who had been sent to the clinic by his wife because she was tired of his irritability. He didn't really want to come to class, but he did his homework and one day returned in wonderment because he noticed how beautiful the moon had been the night before and had taken his wife out to show it to her. A truck driver, large and gruff, told us how he parked his truck at the side of the road at lunchtime to do his body scan. He described being deep into his meditation and feeling some large jolts. While he was focusing on his breath in his body someone had come by and tried to hijack the truck and its contents. As he told the story, he was incredulous rather than enraged, and got us all to laugh. I was impressed.

In class, we focused on process. "This isn't a therapy group," Jon would say if he noticed me slipping into a therapist's role and being seduced by the patient's story, which was usually history.

"Every moment is a fresh moment. Where are you now?" I'd ask class members. In my psychotherapy practice, patients often traced a feeling back to an earlier time, such as a problem with a mother or father or close relative. Together, we investigated it. In class this wasn't relevant unless the experience was actively occurring.

"What are you noticing now?" was a more useful question to be asking. Or, "Can you locate the expression of this feeling in your body? If so, where?" And, "Is this reaction familiar to you? When you notice it, what happens next?"

"How interesting," I might comment.

Class members often questioned the usefulness of bringing attention to the problem and sticking to the present moment. They'd ask, "Why is this helpful?" Then I'd use the model created by Gary Schwartz from the University of Arizona. Schwartz talked about the body's need to maintain a sense of homeostasis. To do this, he said, one must have an intention to pay attention. If not . . . .

dis-attention ➞ **dis-connection** ➞ **dis-regulation** ➞
dis-order ➞ **dis-ease**

I drew this on the board and then I erased the dis's to show how

intention ➞ **attention** ➞ **connection** ➞
regulation ➞ **order** ➞ **ease**

I'd often give the example of my husband, David. "He's a physician," I'd say, "and he ignores his body and doesn't eat lunch, then he wonders why he gets irritable." I then told the class how after I suggested (nagged) him to eat he noticed he had more energy and was less irritable. The class would laugh and I'd feel good that I had demonstrated my point until one day in my meditation it occurred to me that it wasn't very skillful or nice to use my husband as a bad example. It didn't reflect well on either of us.

I had met David during the period when my mother was dying from lung cancer. I had been teaching in the Stress Reduction Program for two years and was continuing to study with Larry and go on retreats. My proclivity to choose boyfriends who weren't particularly nice to me was becoming clear under the heat of awareness. My mother's illness had turned up the heat in my life and I was burning and bubbling away with sadness and fear. I wasn't ready for her to die. I commuted from Cambridge to Mt. Vernon to be with her. She had just turned 70 and was fighting for her life. She felt very weak and was afraid. To ease her pain, I sat and breathed with her, calmly matching my words of comfort and instruction to her breath.

"Breathing in, calming," I'd say to her. "Breathing out, relaxing, and releasing any worries and fears." I'd see her breathing slow down and I felt her calming. She'd then hold my hand and talk to me releasing fears and worries, and I'd listen. Then I would turn on the body scan tape that I had with me and do my own calming. Sadness would arise and I'd do my best to breathe with it as my eyes teared and I prepared myself to say good-bye to her. Mom only lived about five months after she was diagnosed, but she kept the tape I made for her beside her bed and listened to it every night. It comforted her and helped her sleep. She had a massive stroke before she died and lost her cognition, but the beauty of her smile remained. It was the smile of a young girl, trusting and innocent. It helped me see that she was no longer her body, although the body that contained her held on for two weeks after the stroke and it was painful to visit her in the hospital and see her disrobed, discolored, and clearly physically uncomfortable.

During this period I was dating David, as well as a neighbor in Cambridge. Each morning I'd get up at 5 A.M. and go to the Meditation Center in Cambridge. The discipline of meditation and the safety of the retreat center held and supported me. I followed my breath and my mind would obsess on the two men I was dating. Who should I marry? Bringing my attention back to my breath, I did my best to allow my different feelings to flow through. It helped me steady and continue to teach, even though I was upset and sad.

After Mom died David came to the funeral. My mother hadn't met him. She was too sick. When I told her I had met a Jewish doctor, she had said, "I can't meet anyone else. Your neighbor is nice. You'll be all right."

This hurt. I wanted her to be proud of me. At last, at the age of 42, I was with someone I knew she'd approve of as a husband for me. I wanted to make her happy. I felt she had given up on my ability to settle down and be in a lasting relationship. I couldn't accept that she didn't want to meet him.

David, who had never met any of my family, came to her funeral out of respect and to support me. It was comforting to have him beside me. His tenderness and thoughtfulness won me over. No other boyfriend had been so considerate of my needs. As an added bonus, he was tall and I thought he was good looking. If we had kids, they wouldn't have to be short, like me.

I was waking up. Maybe meditation was helping me see more clearly and helping me make better choices. In 1986, six months after my mother died, David and I got married. My father walked me down the aisle. My niece, Anna, was our flower girl. I wore my aunt's wedding dress and my mother-in-law-to-be helped me fasten it.

Breathing in, I calm. Breathing out, I smile.
Each moment is a precious moment.

I hoped to have children with David, but it was not to be. I had waited too long. After a laparoscopy, surgery for pelvic adhesions, two ectopic pregnancies, and a failed in-vitro fertilization, at the age of 45, I decided it was time to stop trying to conceive a biological child. If a child had been placed on our doorstep we might have adopted, but we really didn't have the energy or motivation to engage in that process. Trying to have a baby put some strain on our relationship. We needed to shift focus.

Around that time I heard of Thich Nhat Hahn, a Vietnamese monk who had a retreat center in the south of France. Going there sounded like a wonderful way for me to replenish and recover from my failed pregnancies. Thich Nhat Hahn talks about smiling *into* your sorrow. I wanted to experience his peace in the face of the tragedy of Vietnam. I needed to make peace with my losses.

BODY SCAN MEDITATION

Meditation is about being present in body and mind. Bringing awareness to our body is a powerful exercise in awareness. The body is our foundation. Without it there would be no thought, no breath and no ability to use our sense organs to experience life. Often there is an aversion to being in our body, especially if we are experiencing pain or discomfort, mental or physical. Paradoxically, the more we are able to be in our body, with the intention to observe and be with the sensation, rather than resist it, the easier it is to cope with thoughts, feelings and physical sensations. By simply observing and allowing, we are working with ourselves, rather than resisting what is beyond our ability to control. The more we can observe what arises, with compassion and care, the easier it is to be at home and relaxed with our set of circumstances.

TO DO THE BODY SCAN it is best to get into a comfortable position, either lying down with your arms alongside your body, or sitting in a comfortable chair, preferably a recliner. As with other meditations it is important to do this in an environment that is protected and quiet and will support your ability to relax. It can be useful to have a blanket handy should you feel cool as you engage in this meditation. Make sure you will not be interrupted. Carving time to be by yourself and with yourself is important. This is a time for you, to nurture and care for yourself.

To start, bring your awareness to your breath and let it rest in an area where it is easy to observe its effect on the body. If you like, you can rest your hand on your belly, imagining the belly is like a balloon filling with air and rising on the in-breath and falling, like a balloon deflating, on the out-breath. Simply notice, do not try to change your breath in any way, but bring awareness to the motion of breathing with kindness and compassion. You can note whether the breath is slow or fast, even or irregular. Remember not to judge what is happening, simply observe.

As you're ready, you can let your eyes close and mentally sweep through the body. Let yourself experience the body as a whole, noticing if there are any particular areas that are sensitive. Notice if there is any resistance to doing this. Are there parts of the body you can feel easily and others that are barely discernible? Are you experiencing any sensations you wish would go away? Let yourself be aware of these sensations and do your best to open to your experience, whatever it is. When you do this you can notice when you want to push away or close down, as well as when you want to linger longer. When your attention wanders, simply notice, and bring it gently but firmly back into your body.

If you like, you can imagine your breath traveling down from its entry point into the body down into your extremities. Beginning on the left side, let your awareness move down the body into your foot on the left side. If you are short for time you can do both feet together. However, do not rush this process. The more carefully you can bring awareness into your body parts, the more precise your attention will be. Slowly, connect to your feet, beginning with the toes, moving into the heel, the soles of your feet, the arch and top of the foot. When you feel that you have observed it fully, let the foot dissolve in your awareness and move into the ankle.

If you are not experiencing any sensation in a particular part, simply note it. If there is a vivid experience in another area of the body, you can bring your attention to it and then when you are ready, you can let it go and return to where you were. Simply notice and if you like, breathe with the sensation as best you can. What do you notice about it?

Repeat this process through your body, first the left side and then the right. Moving from the foot into:

Ankle ➝ Lower Leg ➝
Knee ➝ Upper Leg ➝
Hip Bones ➝ Pelvis ➝ Buttocks ➝ Spine ➝
Lower back ➝ Middle back ➝ Upper back ➝

Shoulders ➤ Upper Arm ➤ Elbow ➤ Lower Arm ➤
Wrist ➤ Hand ➤ Finger tips ➤
Abdomen ➤ Diaphragm ➤ Chest ➤
Throat ➤ Neck ➤ Head
(Begin with the jaw and move up through the mouth, ears,
nose, eyes, eyebrows and between the eyebrows,
the forehead and into the scalp.)

Let yourself rest in the sensations of the moment, releasing tension and worries with the out breath and bringing vitality and renewal with the in-breath. If you like, when you have finished scanning the body you can imagine an opening at the crown of the head through which energy enters, and imagine this energy traveling through the body as a whole. You can send energy with your mind to any area that needs special attention, caressing it with the breath. The energy can move in through the crown of your head and leave through the soles of your feet and then enter again in through the soles of your feet and up through the entire body, releasing at the crown of the head.

You may do this as may times as you like, knowing that each time you do this body scan you are taking an active part in your own wellness.

EXERCISE: WHAT'S COOKING?

*This is a good time to review your goals
and your contract with yourself.*

GET INTO YOUR MEDITATION position, take some breaths and settle in.

Now ask yourself, *"What is my commitment to myself?"*

Let this question sink in, asking it again and again, as if you're throwing a pebble deep down through the surface of a pond, going deeper and deeper so it is untouched by any storm. Let this pebble sink down until it reaches the bottom where it can settle and be still.

Allow your deepest desire for freedom and peace to come to you. Commit yourself to it, write it down, and let it guide your actions. How does it affect your ability to: be happy, work with sorrow, maintain a state of equanimity?

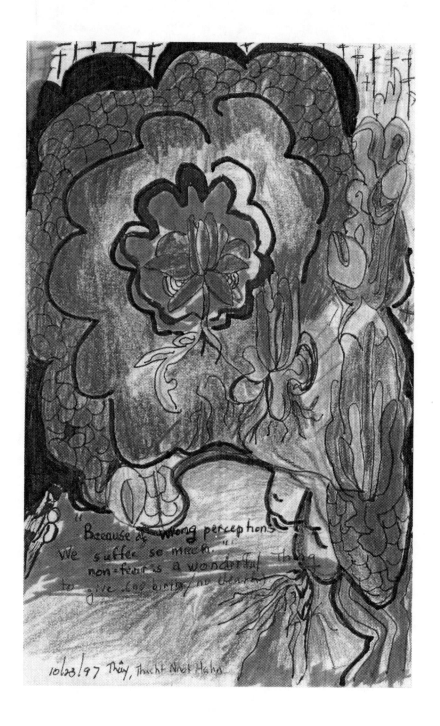

TURNING GARBAGE INTO ROSES

For Warmth
I hold my face between my hands
No, I am not crying.
I hold my face between my hands
to keep my loneliness warm
two hands protecting
two hands nourishing
two hands to prevent
my soul from leaving me
in anger.

— *Zen Poems*, Nhat Hanh

Loss is inevitable but unhappiness is not. My mind knows this but it tends to linger on unhappiness rather than joy. It's expressed in my body with a heaviness in my chest around the area of my heart, a constriction in my throat and a lethargy of spirit.

Everything is always changing; there is life and there is death. Some things are not meant to be but others are. Could I open to the truth and use my pain as transformation to grow larger, wiser, and stronger when I realized I could never have a biological child? I had tried so hard, and waited so long for conditions to be right, and it was too late. I wondered how Thich Nhat Hahn maintained his equanimity after personally witnessing the tragedy of the civil war that tore apart his homeland, Vietnam, and spewed forth other atrocities such as the boat people and the rape and pillage of innocents.

Each difficult moment has the potential
to open my eyes and open my heart.
— Myla Kabat-Zinn

I had no idea at this time that my response to this loss might help prepare the way for my response seven years later when I was diagnosed with lymphoma. I did know I wanted to move through my sadness and be in harmony in body, mind and spirit.

Every year I go on retreat for at least ten days. I also love to travel. It wakes up my senses and refreshes my spirit. Plum Village in the countryside in the south of France in the Dordogne Region meets both criteria. It is in a beautiful location hidden away in an ancient village, nestled among vineyards and farmland. It is also a refuge for Vietnamese who want to maintain their culture and faith. It seemed like the perfect place to recover and renew.

At Plum Village, I discovered that I had brought my feelings of hurt and loss with me. Children flocked around *Thay*, the Vietnamese title for teacher, which is what everyone affectionately calls Thich Nhat Hahn. I watched, jealous, as he walked hand-in-hand with children throughout the day. He could be seen laughing with them and teaching them how to stop and notice the wonders of a leafy tree or a bird in a nest, a flower, or a small ant. When we did a walking meditation, he led it with a child on either side of him. They laughed, he laughed. I felt sad.

"Practice begins in the home," he'd say in talk after talk, as he encouraged the whole family to meditate together. I wished I had a family. A few friends were there with their children and I envied them.

The children sat in the first few rows in the meditation hall and I sat right behind them, feeling the pang in my heart and the disappointment in my head at not having my own child. My mind was filled with longing. There was no fleeing the storm of pain and disappointment I felt in being barren. Yet, as Thay softly spoke about planting seeds of mindfulness and compassion, and as I slowly paid attention, washing the dishes with a rubber hose over the drain outside the kitchen area, or making my bed on the foam pad that rested on the floor in an old stone farmhouse, or talking with other people from Europe, Asia, and the United States, I began to open like the flowers that Thay talked about growing and being fertilized by the compost heap. My concentration increased and I began to focus more on what was occurring, rather than what was not. There was a richness of sense impressions, which Thay pointed out daily. There were trees and flowers, a flowing river, exotic tastes of Vietnamese food and smells.

The bathrooms couldn't hold all that was being released by us yogis and the cesspool overflowed, adding to the richness of aromas surrounding us. It seemed that we were all letting go so much that collectively we clogged up the septic system and help had to be called in to flush it out. I imagined all the French soil that we might be fertilizing. Was this a lesson? A metaphor for what we were doing?

Muscular French men arrived with high black boots and giant vacuum tubes to suction out the clogged pipes. On our way to the meditation hall, we stopped to watch them, impressed and relieved. We were certainly returning to basics. How mindful and calm were we as we waited in long lines to use the few working toilets?

As I let myself be involved and absorbed by the daily life of the village, my awareness expanded and I began to take pleasure from having the children around. I realized that my life need not be empty of their joy. Everyone had lost something or had been unhappy about something. I was not the only one practicing smiling into my pain as Thay suggested.

My connection with the others at Plum Village — monks and nuns, Westerners from the United States and Europe, the Vietnamese, old and young and in between — and our connection with each other, our connection to the earth, our feet touching the soil, our noses breathing in the sweet scent of flowers and the rancid smell of the septic system, our eyes gazing beyond the hamlet over vineyards and farms, our ears hearing birdsong and flute music and Thay's words about his pain and the compassion it evoked, all helped me bear my own pain. I began to heal.

When I went to Plum Village for a second time a few years later, I learned more about the need to let go and travel light. I arrived in Paris on my way to Plum Village following a vacation in Israel with my husband, David. David left me in Tel Aviv to return to Boston and to work. I had two more days in Israel and then planned to go on to France. In preparation, the day before I left I made a special trip to the airport in Tel Aviv to ship my bags. I hoped this would save time and avoid possible confusion at the airport the next day. All went smoothly, but when I arrived at Charles DeGaulle Airport in Paris, I learned that my bags had not made the trip with me. They had been sent ahead to New York, which was my destination after Plum Village.

When I left Tel Aviv the weather had been very hot and humid. In Paris it was cold and damp. I had only the clothes on my back: shorts, a halter top, a blouse and sandals. I was cold, tired, and couldn't speak French. I found an English-speaking airline official who assured me that my bags would be located and sent to Plum Village. Everyone was quite nice and I was given fifty dollars, a small comb, a toothbrush, and a small tube of toothpaste to tide me over until my luggage arrived. I bought sweatpants and a matching sweatshirt, underwear and a pair of socks. I left Paris feeling light and unencumbered as I made the trip by train to Plum Village.

Plum Village has two hamlets, one high, overlooking vineyards, and one low, more like a delta with a river running through it. When I arrived it had been raining and the ground was very muddy and soggy. I was assigned to a room in the lower hamlet, in a barracks-like building. One side of the barracks had rooms and the other side contained the showers for the entire hamlet. It was wet — very wet. There was no escape from the mud or the dampness. I did not have a car and there was no easy transportation out. There was only one telephone in the whole lower hamlet. Because I needed to contact the airlines to see if my suitcase had arrived, and since I couldn't speak French, I always had to find a French-speaking person to help me call the airline. Getting through to the right department and person was frustrating. It took a long time and was often unsuccessful. I was cold and I WANTED my clothes.

One friend loaned me his jacket. Another, a tall woman, lent me her nightshirt, which I wore as a dress. Days passed and not only did my suitcase not arrive, but it was very difficult to track and to get through to the proper authorities. Depending totally on others, even to make telephone calls, was challenging and frustrating. Locating my luggage became a major task. Meanwhile, the sun of southern France was not shining, the cold, damp weather continued, and it was still raining almost every day. My sandals, my sweatsuit and my one pair of socks were becoming muddier and muddier as I literally chilled out. My mantra at the time was, "Let Go."

A friend, thinking he'd help, told me an old Zen story about a farmer who was distraught because he had lost his cows. While he was out looking for them he met a monk. The monk, seeing he is upset, asks if he can help. He learns that the farmer cannot return to his village without his cows. The two continue looking for the animals without success. The farmer is miserable, but the monk has no cows to lose or to locate. He is free to move on.

In the mud, squishing along, fed by the compassion of my friends' loaning me their shirts, their time, and their warmth, I, too, began to let go and move on, feeling lighter and freer than I had in years. No need now to dress up. Navy blue, the color of my sweatsuit, was very unflattering. No need to look pretty. And I began to enjoy the freedom of not having to maintain any facade. No cows. No decisions about what to wear. If the weather warmed, I had my shorts. If it was cold, I wore my sweatsuit. When we finally did go to the train station in Bergerac to claim my luggage, half of it had been stolen . . . and I could smile. Less to carry.

EXERCISE: LETTING GO

Find a coin or piece of jewelry and put it in the palm of your hand. Now close your fingers around it and feel it in your hand. Hold on to it as tight as you can, really grasping it. Can you bring attention to the physical sensations of doing this? Can you notice your breathing? Do you notice any particular mental states or emotions? When you feel you've grasped it long enough, let it go. What happens? What physical sensations, thoughts or feelings do you notice? Does your breathing change as you do this? Simply observe.

Now, turn your hand over and hold the item you have selected lightly in the center of your hand, palm upright, fingers relaxed, the hand open, parallel to the floor. What does it feel like now, to be holding the item lightly in an open palm?

Can you think of any desire or disappointment that you've been holding on to very tightly? What would happen if you held it more lightly or let go of it entirely? Is there any garbage that you are holding on to that you'd like to release and convert into fertilizer? Can you imagine what flowers or fruit might grow if you did this?

If you choose to do so, make a list, *simply observing without judgment* what you'd release.

DAD AND THE FIVE REMEMBRANCES

I am sure to grow old.
I can not avoid aging.

I am sure to become sick.
I can not avoid sickness.

I am sure to die.
I can not avoid death.

All things dear and beloved to me
are subject to change and separation.

I am the owner of my actions;
I will become the heir of my actions.

— Anguttara Nikaya

My father, "smilin' Jack" Rosenbaum, never meditated or heard Thich Nhat Hahn say, "Breathing in I calm, Breathing out I smile." However, Dad smiled frequently and naturally, even after he was diagnosed with mesothelioma, cancer of the lining of the abdomen. Somehow he could see the glass half full as opposed to half empty. He wasn't daunted by his diminished strength or the need to move from his apartment in Mt. Vernon, New York, where he was born and had lived 79 years.

My father cheerfully moved into our house in Worcester, leaving behind lifelong friends, neighbors, the bagel man, and a girlfriend. He brought some clothes, colorful ties, some hats, art supplies, photographs and a certificate of appreciation from the Mt. Vernon School System. He also brought get-well cards from the fifth graders he had entertained and charmed by telling stories and reading to them. They were addressed to *Grandpa Jack Rosenbaum* and were now tacked to the wall in his bedroom.

His room, off our kitchen, was now his home, and like his old home office, was filled with clutter, all recently acquired. There were old newspapers, which he saved to cut out coupons, notepads, letters, and books. Outside the window by his bed he had us erect a bird feeder. He'd lie in bed and gaze out the window, taking pleasure from watching the birds and inventing new ways to keep the squirrels at bay. On the wall was a card he had made that said:

In order to get to the other side
you must leave the shore.

How wonderful. How excited he felt to be alive for another day. Every morning he'd greet me as I came downstairs towards his room by calling my name, "ELANA!"

I'd open the door of his room and he'd be lying in bed with a big smile on his face and proclaim "I'M HERE!" He made sure each day to say, "I love you."

I told my Stress Reduction classes stories about my father. It impressed me that he seemed so alive and fully engaged in life. He even made new friends at a group for senior Jewish men. His joy, his ability to be present, his love and lack of fear at facing death inspired me.

Yet, my ability to appreciate my father and his zest for living and loving didn't happen immediately. There was "old stuff" I needed to release first. So many of his characteristics — his impracticality, sentimentality, *schmaltziness*, his need to please — were hard for me to accept. I recognized these traits in myself and didn't like them. I often felt he needed to be the center of attention and everyone else (me) had to take a back seat. Dad was very loving, but he also could be very embarrassing and demanding. In restaurants I noticed myself holding my breath and wanting to flee into the bathroom when the soup he'd ordered arrived at the table. He always ordered hot soup, "very hot," he'd say. If it arrived lukewarm he'd scowl at the waiter or waitress and yell, "I ordered it hot! HOT! BRING IT BACK!"

When he was uncomfortable and in pain it was hard for me. He rarely complained, but at times, especially when being sick was new to him, he'd get very irritable and take it out on me, criticizing me or finding fault with something I did. To continue to care for him, I found that I needed to be assertive. One day when I came home from work, Dad was uncomfortable and particularly irritable. Nothing I could do was right. The more I tried, the worse it became. Finally, I sat down next to him on the bed and took his hand. "Tell me what's bothering you," I said. "I'm not leaving until you do."

"Nothing . . . leave me alone."

Stubbornly I remained, not letting go of his hand.

Dad continued to yell at me.

I sat there quietly. He kept yelling at me, " I told you to leave!"

My temper rose, but in control I said, "Stop, I will not tolerate this nastiness."

I continued to sit, holding his hand, consciously following my breath and noticing as my heart rate began to accelerate. My jaw was set. I was not leaving until we had an understanding. We were at an impasse.

The silence grew.

Dad started crying. He said he was afraid. Suddenly my perception shifted. The tightness in my body eased as I saw and felt his vulnerability. My genuine compassion and love went out to him and my anger dissolved. Then I could hold him, say "I love you," and comfort him.

Now I could trust his "thank you" and "I love you." I could even smile when he'd pull me in his room and tell me, "Be nice to David," whom he held in high esteem. The encounter was healing for both of us. It enabled me to listen and see more clearly the love and sweetness of this man, my father. Loving him helped me love myself.

Dad spent his last few months with my brother Bob and his family, my nieces, Anna and Bekka, and Judi, Bob's wife. He loved California and the Bay area where Bob lived and had hoped to spend

the winter in this warmer climate, enjoy San Francisco, and then
return to Worcester, where he had been for the past year and a half.
Instead, he grew steadily weaker. Knowing he was failing, David and
I traveled to California to be with him again.

It was January 18, 1995, my brother's birthday. David had just
returned home to Massachusetts and Bob had taken the day off from
work. He and I were sitting and meditating by Dad's bedside as his
breath became shallow. We heard the rattle of his labored breathing
and then there was silence. I opened my eyes and Dad's arm moved.
Bob was still sitting. I closed my eyes again. The silence filled the
room. Breath did not return.

My father had wanted to live fully until the end. Just the night
before, he, who almost never drank alcohol, had asked my husband
for a beer and instructed him how to pour it so that it would have a
head. It was important that it be just so. We couldn't find beer in the
house so David substituted root beer. Dad, the paint salesman, who
loved color, form, and taste, wasn't fooled. He, who was alive to new
experiences, saw even the pouring and sipping of a beer as an adventure.
He liked the taste, but he loved the froth. Later that night I wrote in
my journal.

We love you, Jack.
We love you, Grandpa.
We love you, Daddy.

Then I jotted down what he had said to me and lived throughout
my life and his.

Life is an adventure . . .
Experience with all your senses . . .
Enjoy . . . Smile.

Bob and I continued to sit a few minutes longer by Dad's side
until the doorbell rang and the hospice nurse entered. She went over
to Dad and said, "He's not breathing." I told her it was my brother's
birthday and she said, "How wonderful; my mother died on my
birthday." Only now can I appreciate what she meant. Life continues.
My father had died, but life continues. It continues in us.

My father had been wearing a t-shirt I had given him from our synagogue in Worcester. It showed a *lulav shake*, promoting the celebration of the holiday of Succoth, when you shake a *lulav*, a palm frond, to the four directions and in an upward motion toward the sky and down toward the earth. This represents unity and shows that God is everywhere. Emma, the hospice nurse, cleaned off the shirt and washed off the dried blood that was caked on his arms and in the crevice of his collarbone. She washed his goatee and combed his hair and covered him up with a lovely quilt. It was reassuring and comforting. Life does go on.

Bob and I sat with Dad again, this time in silence, breathing and guiding Dad's spirit. Filled with love and peace we said good-bye.

Later, my niece, Bekka, came home and we all sat quietly together by Grandpa. After he was taken to the funeral home, Bekka, Bob, and I went to pick up Anna, who was 15, at her school. Bekka asked me why I wanted to go.

"To see life," I said.

Puzzled, Bekka responded, "But life is here."

On the way home Bekka turned to me and asked, "Enough life?" And in my journal I wrote:

> *Enough life? Who knows?*
> *I do know I'm going to give it my all to make it so.*

Then I jotted down a little poem.

> *air*
> *the*
> *in   one needs-*
> *up   an open heart,*
> *fly   love,*
> *to   trust.*
> *   and to be able to smile.*

Thank you, Dad, for teaching me to smile, to trust, to soar, and to live life and whatever it brings as an adventure, to see the beauty and the good that is here.

And three months later I discovered I had cancer.

GUIDED MEDITATION ON DYING

Take a moment to reflect on what you have just read. See if you can bring awareness to any sensations in the body, letting your attention rest on the rhythm of your breath, a reminder that you are here now, giving yourself this time to reflect on death and its meaning to you.

Simply notice what arises as you allow the awareness of death to be present. You may do this meditation with your eyes open or closed, whatever helps you access this experience with greater depth. As you do so, bringing attention to the breath grounds you, calming mind and body, and supports you so you can observe what arises, as if you were sitting in an easy chair observing a show.

As you bring attention to your breathing, you can let into your awareness the sense of someone in your life who has died, letting this person, and the experience of his or her death, come to you. How old were you at the time? What was your relationship to this person? Notice any feelings or thoughts that you may have as you allow this experience to come. Does this in any way inform your expectations about your own death? Does it influence how you are living now? In what way?

When you are ready, open your eyes and jot down any words or thoughts that express what you have just experienced. You may also choose to do this exercise non-verbally, using color and form and choosing any art material — clay, paint, colored pencils, crayons, or pastels — that feels comfortable. You could also choose to create a collage that represents the different elements of this experience. Simply notice what arises and breathe into it with love.

SECTION II

Everything Changes

It was March of 1995. I was sitting in a bookstore cafe with my friend Ruth who is a psychiatrist. Ruth was directly across from me, and as we were talking she asked, "Has your face always been asymmetrical?"

"No," I said. "It hasn't."

I had noticed some fullness on one side, but looking in the mirror I had just attributed it to getting plumper and perimenopausal weight gain. Now I wondered.

My husband David is a primary care physician. He was also in the bookstore. Spotting him, I yelled across the aisles, "DAVID!" Sweet man that he is, David came over to our table right away and hearing Ruth's question he felt my neck . . . and got very quiet. There was a lump. Concerned, he arranged for me to see an ENT physician the very next day to do a needle biopsy. The young doctor reassured me it was probably nothing. This was a Friday. I wouldn't get the results until Monday.

I remember going to the Bar Mitzvah of a friend's son over the weekend and whispering to another friend, also a physician, that I was worried. I had her feel my lump.

She, too, reassured me. Maybe the lump was an infected salivary duct. "This often happens," she said.

On Monday, the biopsy showed that the lump was malignant. I got the news by phone right after my stress reduction class. I was in the middle of a meeting with the interns who had been observing my class so that they could teach MBSR. I felt numb, in shock. How could this be? I had taken care of myself, I meditated, ate right, had loving relationships and meaningful work.

My first impulse was to search my mind for reasons why this could have happened. I know the mind affects the body, but I do not believe that I did this to myself. There were periods in my life when I had been depressed, but it was in the past. Maybe I had a genetic pre-disposition to cancer. My mother died of lung cancer when she was 70; my father, of mesothelioma.

There was no way to know the cause, I reminded myself. Things happen. I told myself that I'd done nothing wrong, but some doubt lingered. Had I done my best? Had my tendency to get depressed lowered my immune system? My father had just died a few months earlier. I had enjoyed having him with us the last year of his life, but had it unconsciously predisposed me to cancer?

I had a CAT scan and another tumor was discovered in the right pelvic area. I was diagnosed with stage three non-Hodgkin's lymphoma. I would need chemotherapy. The cancerous cells were not growing quickly, but they were advancing. This cancer was in the lymph system and could travel through the body and reside in any organ. The type I had was a mixed cell variety, large and small cells, low to intermediate grade. I was slated to have a minimum of six treatments about three weeks apart, depending on how well my body responded to the chemotherapy.

I was dazed and overwhelmed with information. When I looked in the mirror, I no longer thought, "I'm getting plump," but "Why didn't I notice this before?" I didn't feel different. I tired easily, but I was also working full time. I taught classes, I had a busy private practice in psychotherapy, and I had been caring for and living with my 80-year-old father, who had just died three months earlier. At 52, I was also getting older, and pre-menopausal.

Everyone around me — family, friends, students, colleagues — was shocked that I had cancer. I was the first one of my generation to have a life-threatening illness. "This too shall pass" was a phrase often used at the clinic, but normally we weren't talking about the fragility of life. My husband sat with me and cried. When I met my friend, Susan, for lunch she cried. I went to the doctor's office later and wrote:

Well, it's been a ride. I sit under the skylight in the clinic waiting to see the nurse for my physical, waiting for my bone marrow biopsy, waiting and breathing, being quiet, in the light. Asking myself daily, hour after hour, minute by minute, "What is important?"

My doctor, Dr. Chris Seidler, just opened the door of the examining room. I breathed in the air and bathed in the sunlight. May that be a metaphor for this experience.

The nurse practitioner was friendly and I got to lie down and calm myself so my appetite returned and I actually got hungry again but I felt headachy and nauseous. The seriousness of this is hitting me.

No, I'm not ready. No, why me?

And sadness comes. Sadness hit when Jennifer, our secretary at work, had to cancel my patients for Wednesday and Thursday and I couldn't tell her when she could reschedule them. When I listened to the panic in Saki's voice: "Jettison the interns who're slated to be in your class." The realization that I may not be able to work makes this diagnosis all too real. CHEMO!

I've already gotten some relaxation tapes of ocean and Bach and Hebrew chants and Hasidic melodies and I plan on getting bright colored scarves for my head — forget the wig.

I want to shout out to everyone, "I have THE BIG C *and I* AM ALIVE! *I am here."*

Yes. BUT. . . .

I don't like this.

I am now waiting for blood tests, x-ray, pre-admission work-up, and then a bone marrow biopsy. I'm calm and disturbed.

"It hurts," says the doctor, as he readies the needle for my bone marrow biopsy. Hurt doesn't bother me. Needing this procedure is what upsets me. I'm finding it difficult to accept this is happening to me.

Present moment; precious moment; I just have to be in it. This is my challenge. I don't have the luxury of NOT being here now if I don't want to suffer.

I feel love.
I feel hope.
I am afraid.

I do not know
Will I survive this horrible, insidious, invisible
Take over of fat hungry cells that destroy the healthy ones?
Bubbles of destruction.

If I could will them away I would.

Anger surfaces.
No!

Go away.
Why me?

Have I surrendered?
Yes. No.

I'd like to wail . . . not fair.
I want to live more.
Splash about. Learn. Explore.

New moment.
It is here.
And still am I.

Guided Meditation: Awareness Of Breathing

Nourishing Mind and Heart Through Awareness

This meditation begins with awareness of the breath. It is designed to help quiet and calm the mind by developing a space inside yourself that is still, where you can feel safe and secure, even in the midst of a life-altering event such as a diagnosis of cancer. As with the other meditations in this book, the attitude that you bring to it is as important as your focus of attention. The more you can see this as an exploration and learning, a time to care for yourself and to nurture yourself, the easier it will be. Simply taking this time will allow you to come to know yourself better and make decisions based on wisdom and hope rather than on fear. Doing this regularly can be a vital complement to any medical treatment and help sustain you in times of change and difficulty.

YOU CAN BEGIN BY NOTICING the way your breath is moving in the body. If you like, you can put your hand on your belly and feel the way it moves with the breath. You may notice that as you breathe in the belly rises . . . and as you breathe out it falls.

If you like, you can imagine that you are breathing in oxygen and nutrients and sending it to all parts of the body . . . and breathing out, releasing, and letting go of any tension. Simply notice the breath as it comes in and as it goes out. Notice the rhythm of the breath, feeling what it's like without trying to alter it in any way. Breathing in, be aware that you're breathing in. Breathing out, be aware that you're breathing out.

There is nothing that you have to do. You can be a witness to any thoughts that come and go in the mind, like watching subtitles on a movie screen, changing as the scenes change, and yet your breath continues flowing in, and out, as the movie goes on. Your breath is also moving and changing, coming and going . . . like a wave of relaxation, bringing in energy and renewal, and then releasing.

As you breathe in, you can imagine that you're boosting healthy cells and bringing in positive energy, and as you breathe out, releasing toxins from the body. You can imagine any destructive cells dissolving and being washed away, flushed out as the breath continues moving in and out, again and again, like the tides of the sea. Let yourself be aware that you're breathing and letting go of everything except your attention to the movement of your breath. Let yourself be receptive to this cleansing process.

You may also be aware of sounds and the experience of sitting or lying still as you rest and bring awareness to the moment, taking this time for yourself, for replenishment and revitalization. As you allow yourself to reside in the moment as you are experiencing it, without trying to change it, you'll be fostering relaxation and calm. You can release more and more as you settle into this moment, softening into it, gently. And letting go of any negativity, letting yourself receive the bounty that is here for you . . . able to discover it more and more as you practice paying attention and as you continue noticing the breath, breathing, and being present, here, right now . . . as fully as you can.

In the silence, in the stillness, let yourself be held, opening to all the people in your life who love you and are caring for you and wishing you well. And you can know that as you do this meditation you are nourishing spirit and mind, head and heart . . . in a continual cycle with each breath, connecting to forces larger than your self.

If you like, you can picture yourself vibrant and whole, enjoying life and fully participating in it, smiling, laughing, opening to new experiences . . . and the wonder of it all . . . being here, now.

THE CHALLENGE AND THE COMMITMENT

The experience of the world is processed
by our minds
Filtered by our experience

What is it that enables us to make connections
creating happiness or sadness?

Perception is my topic
Seeing life's events as a challenge.
Knowing when and of what we have control.
Making wise commitments.

Challenge — Control — Commitment
lend themselves to Stress Hardiness

Courage lets us be free
To hold it all
With love.

My commitment not to suffer and to really welcome each moment as precious presented the biggest challenge of my life. It was truly meditation in action, the fruition of all my retreats and meditations. Could I maintain a sense of equanimity and focus on the present moment, the difficult ones as well as the pleasant?

Discovering I had cancer was such a surprise and a dislocation of routine. My colleagues at the Stress Reduction Clinic were in a state of disbelief. Mindfulness meditation is about impermanence, but now? And to me? I wasn't ready to confront my own mortality so soon.

And others reacted. At the dinner table, my husband would look at me and cry. Friends were supportive but they, too, were disbelieving. Some people didn't know how to respond.

The outpouring of support is almost overwhelming, but David's cousins called and they didn't know what to say. It seems that "cancer" evokes strong feelings of fear and discomfort. I have to deal with the reactions of others as well as myself. Some people feel the need to give advice like, "It's good you went and got a dog . . . You know, mind and spirit go together."

I used everything I could to help me manage the assault of doctors, procedures, and chemotherapy. When I felt really stuck in a feeling, such as sadness or frustration, and no attention to my breath would dispel it, I'd put it on paper either in the form of a poem or images, some of which I've included in this book. This allowed me to move the feeling from inside me to outside. Sometimes just napping or finding a sympathetic ear made a difference.

"Perseverance furthers" was my motto. I'd look at the lithograph I have hanging in my office of a little tugboat, small and chunky, not very glamorous or sleek like the big boats in the harbor (my secret wish is to be tall, slender, wear big hats, and eat as many ice creams as I'd like). I identified with that tugboat. It was sturdy and had a lot of power. It reminded me of *Little Toot*, a children's story I read when I was little. In it, Little Toot plays a lot. He is little and isn't respected, but when a big storm comes and none of the bigger boats can help the grand ocean liner, Little Toot courageously comes to the rescue. He knows how to ride the waves and stay afloat. Seeing this, the big boats stop laughing at him and applaud his bravery.

I'm a little tugboat, stubborn, and determined. I never knew it was a positive trait. I wanted to be a big ocean liner, not five feet tall and insecure. I fought with my mother, the symbol of power in my life. The seas at home were choppy and often high as my parents, too, struggled to stay afloat as caretakers of their own parents. I never knew that my persistence in the face of obstacles would be useful as I battled with cancer and my own ability to ride the waves of a changing mind and body.

When I was little my mother would admonish me, "Stop banging your head against a wall." We never agreed on that wall. I thought she was too fearful; she thought I was impractical, selfish and foolish. The allergist I went to told her she had "Smother love." And I, of course, wanting greater autonomy, agreed.

My mother's relationship to death was quite different from my father's. She didn't see it as an adventure, but was very fearful of it. When she was pre-adolescent, an older sister had been killed in a car accident. As a young mother, four years after I was born she had a second child, Barbara, who was born a "blue baby" with a congenital heart defect. In 1947, surgery for this condition was just being explored. On a hot August day, three days before her scheduled surgery, Barbara died at the age of four and a half months. Mom never really recovered. Less than two years later, my brother Bob was born, but her worries only increased. What if something happened to one of us?

Perhaps my mother's fears and unhappiness motivated me to look more deeply at causality. What does allow for happiness? How do our mental and physical actions affect our well-being? Could I be happy even if my mother could not? I'm sure this contributed to my becoming a therapist and later, a meditator. I wanted to turn my garbage into vegetables and fruit, maybe even flowers.

By simply observing my thought process and not getting lost in it, at least some of the time, I discovered that fear could come AND go; I need not drown in it. As a cancer patient, I knew that my stubbornness and fighting spirit would be useful, but I didn't want to deplete my spirit by fighting what was beyond my ability to control. No more wall banging for me. As Seven of Nine, a Star Trek character, said, "Resistance is futile." I needed to accept what was happening and focus on what was right with me rather than what was wrong.

I could not afford to let my mind run ahead of itself. I concentrated on one session of chemotherapy at a time and tried not to worry about the next one until it was near. There was a new urgency to my practice. I needed to live moment by moment. I was more scared of getting depressed and feeling helpless than I was of cancer.

I've been going over in my mind the sign in the oncology unit here at the hospital that says, "Cancer cannot kill hope; it cannot take away spirit." *I read this when I was here with my father when he was being treated for cancer. At that time I couldn't believe it. I didn't like seeing my Dad become weak. I feared his spirit might be affected. Today I know how true the words are. My spirit is strong. I am alive today. I do not intend to suffer. That is the miracle that my mindfulness meditation practice has given me . . . to be able to appreciate being in the present moment, here now.*

Staying in the moment gave me a sense of control. I could choose how and what to eat; I never lost my appetite, and I was conscious of my nutrition and careful to eat well. Chemotherapy made me hungrier and I gained some weight. I didn't like this, but I decided it was not a time to diet. When I was hungry I fed myself. I appreciated the crackers and hard candies at the oncology office and I'd carry my own healthier treats. I also saw a doctor of herbal medicine and acupuncture. I had massages regularly. I called up people I had known when I lived in Seattle, even my ex-husband, and asked them to pray for me. I had read that this helped.

For years, I talked about stress hardiness in the classes I taught. This is a term that Dr. Suzanne Kobasa coined to describe personality characteristics that seem to protect people from the adverse effects of stress — control, commitment, and challenge. Kobasa found that people who believe that they have some power to influence their lives have a strong sense of control. They are engaged in life and have a strong sense of commitment, energy and enthusiasm for what they do. This control comes not from holding on tight or trying to force something to happen but more from a sense of self-efficacy, an inner knowing and confidence in one's own ability.

Stress causes a fight or flight reaction. I wanted to do both. Could my challenge to myself to be well and free of suffering be strong enough to keep me going? Could I maintain my commitment to being well and fortify my sense of control even with my vulnerability so clear? It seemed that each day brought a new challenge. It was very disturbing to wake up in the morning and find clumps of hair on my pillow, or to fish large masses of it out from the shower drain, but that is what was happening. I couldn't change it.

Tonight I tried on a scarf and considered doffing my glasses and wearing my contact lenses until I learned that my eyes would dry out from the chemotherapy. I'm realizing I'm vain but I don't want to wear a wig, it's not 'me.' People are giving me scarves and I'm giving myself brightly colored ones. I wear them like a turban or draped dramatically. They keep my head warmer.

I was motivated to go deeper down to find what was real and could sustain me. I re-read inspirational books and thought often of the quote I used in my classes from the book *Man's Search for Meaning*, by Victor Frankl. He writes:

> We who lived in concentration camps can remember the men who walked through the huts comforting others, giving away their last piece of bread. They may have been few in number, but they offer sufficient proof that everything can be taken from a man but one thing: the last of the human freedoms — to choose one's attitude in any given set of circumstances.

I'd like to be free of cancer, but that is not within my control. The way I approach this time is under my control. It's important to me to free myself from that which binds and perpetuates suffering. I hope to be free to see clearly, to experience happiness and well being and to face what arises with courage and faith. The present moment is my home. The more I can be HERE with acceptance, the happier I can be.

Last night I went to my Rosh Hodesh group, which in Hebrew means "head of the month," the time of the New Moon. A modern custom among Jewish woman is to come together and study at this time. I normally find my Rosh Hodesh group stimulating and supportive but tonight when I was talking and reflecting on the fact that I didn't know whether I would be here five years from now, one of the members said, "Stop . . . I can't take this anymore."

Her mother died of breast cancer and her sister now had breast cancer, a recurrence. She couldn't tolerate hearing me bring up the fact that I didn't know how long I had to live.

At that moment I realized that I wasn't afraid of dying and I was committed to facing what was happening to me, opening up to it rather than running away. At the same time, I realized that it was she who was suffering, not I. Everything changes and is subject to separation and impermanence. This means me, too. Living and dying are part of the nature of things. The more I can really open to this reality the happier I can be. Is this what non-clinging is about, not holding on to what used to be?

When I went for my first treatment of chemotherapy, I was ushered into a small room that had a bed and a recliner. I was alone and I remember the room as stark and overly bright. I asked the nurse to turn off the fluorescent light and replace it with an incandescent one. Knowing this was my first treatment, she humored me and began searching for another light. The only one she could find was an emergency lamp that ran on batteries. She plugged it in, turned it on for me and turned off the overhead. I laid back in the bed (this first chemotherapy was the only time I got the bed) and listened to my relaxation tape and some music on the Walkman I had brought with me. I remember being very upset that the atmosphere wasn't more soothing. My fuss over the lighting helped me feel more in control. I could not admit to myself I was scared.

I am living moment by moment. This helps. Now I am alive and with friends. I am here . . . and I intend to be here as much as I can.

It was helpful for me to learn more about lymphoma and its treatment. I didn't concentrate on prognosis; too much was unknown. I got on the Internet, had my oncologist send me articles on lymphoma and had a consult with another oncology team in a second hospital, which thankfully confirmed the treatment I was receiving. In addition, I talked to myself: "Things happen . . . Everyone gets sick at some point and dies . . . cancer is what's happening now, use it, learn from it, you don't have to like it . . . you're still here."

When I went for an appointment or chemotherapy, I brought a tape recorder and a tape of music or meditation, a book to read and my journal and colored pencils. I talked to people. I made myself as comfortable as I could and tried my best to continue living my life as before treatment. Of course, this was impossible.

There was much I couldn't control. I never quite knew how I'd respond to chemo. This made planning difficult. My life was busy. I worked at the Stress Reduction Clinic three days a week and saw clients the other two days. I also felt responsible for our meals at home and household chores. I remember lying down during teachers' meetings and forcing myself to stay awake. It didn't make sense. I had to give myself more space to rest. I needed to let go, but I'm proud. I didn't want to cut back at work. Who I was seemed very connected to what I did. Could I still feel worthy if I worked less? I wasn't ready to let go and stop working. Yet, I was committed to maintaining a sense of wellness. That was hard to do if I was exhausted. Where was the balance?

I remembered a story I had heard about a monk who is being chased by a tiger. He runs as fast as he can until he comes to the edge of the cliff. Looking down, he sees a sheer drop down onto ragged rocks below. Looking behind him, he sees the tiger rapidly approaching. He notices a vine growing from the side of the cliff. He takes a leap and grabs onto the vine only to notice a rat gnawing away at it. On the land the tiger is waiting. Down below are the rocks. He looks about and sees a lush, juicy, ripe strawberry nearby. With one hand, he reaches out, plucks it, puts it in his mouth and says, "Delicious."

Being very sick is a little like hanging over a cliff, clutching a precarious vine. Would I be able to have the equanimity and the presence of mind to notice the strawberry, taste it and experience its juicy sweet flavor?

The CAT scans, blood tests and other technological procedures the doctors requested seemed endless. As these large machines descended down on me, I would begin bringing my attention to my breath. I could surrender and calm during these tests but I didn't like having my life interrupted and not knowing what would be.

"Powerful learning," I'd say to myself again and again, as I observed my desire to keep things as they had been, rather than let go and accommodate to how they were now.

Again and again, I'd repeat to myself:

> *Breathing in I calm,*
> *Breathing out I smile.*
> *Dwelling in the present moment,*
> *It is the only moment.*

I tried to remember to forgive myself and be more compassionate towards my own struggles, rooting myself on.

YOU CAN DO IT. YES, YOU CAN.

EXERCISE: STRESS, PERCEPTION, AND DEMANDS

Hans Selye, the father of research on stress, dedicated his book, *Stress*, "To all those who are not afraid to enjoy the stress of a full life, nor so naïve as to think they can do so without intellectual effort." Selye defined stress as, "wear and tear" and "the body's non-specific reaction to a demand." Richard Lazarus, a psychologist, looked at the psychology of stress and defined it as, "The body's response to a demand which it perceives as overwhelming his or her resources." The key words here are 'demand' and 'perceive.'

TAKE A MOMENT to quickly jot down some of the stresses that you currently perceive to be in your life. When you have completed the list, take a few breaths and read it slowly, stopping after each stressor and repeating it to yourself for three breaths, simply noticing what arises in body and in mind.

After you have done this, you may want to ask yourself, *"What is the demand? What are my expectations?"* Let the questions and your response to them reside in your awareness for a few breaths and then write down what came to mind. When you feel ready, move onto the next stressor. It is recommended that you only do one at a time.

When you are finished you can re-read the list and what you have written. Do you notice any similarities in the demands you are placing on yourself? What is under your control to change, what is not? Take your time in answering these questions and return to your breath, following the inhalation and exhalation any time you notice yourself tensing or tightening.

You may answer these questions and do this exercise more than once, noticing how your perception of stress changes.

My stressor is: _____

Its demands are: _____

_____

My expectations are: _____

My stressor is: _____

Its demands are: _____

_____

My expectations are: _____

My stressor is: _____

Its demands are: _____

_____

My expectations are: _____

My stressor is: _____

Its demands are: _____

_____

My expectations are: _____

Now return to your list of stresses. As you read them, what aspects of yourself and your perception of life do they challenge? How could you use this challenge for growth? What parts of you could they strengthen or develop?

If you observe a glass of water filled to the middle, do you see it as half full or half empty or both? It's all in the perspective. What is yours? How does this influence you, if at all, in your response to the above exercises?

What is your commitment to yourself? Write it down.

How does this inform the way you respond to stress? How does it influence the way you are living now?

EXERCISE: WHO AM I?

So often our concept of our self is fixed. I am a woman, or I am a wife, or I am a sister and a stress reduction teacher. But what does that really mean? Everything changes including who we think we are and what defines us. Am I now a cancer patient? What does that mean? Who is Elana? Who do you *think* you are?

FOR THIS EXERCISE, return to your breath, let the mind quiet, and simply ask yourself, *"Who am I?"*

As an answer comes to you ask again, *"Who is that?"*

You can do this with yourself or with another person, taking turns listening and witnessing what arises. Allow responses to come to you; take your time, and pause between responses.

Notice what happens in your body. Let yourself be open to any surprises that enter your awareness without judging what occurs or censoring any thoughts. **Simply notice.**

You can return to your breath anytime you need to steady your attention and be present to the moment as it is **now.**

ON RETREAT: WORKING WITH MIND STATES

How I do love to go up in a swing
Up in the air so high
Then I can see so far and clear
All of the countryside.
And when I go down again
I hang unto the sides
I know I will go up again
And get to enjoy the ride.

— adapted from *The Swing*
Robert Lewis Stevenson

Treatment for cancer takes time, and the mind and body need nourishment, rest and support. After five treatments of chemotherapy and prior to a new CAT scan to determine how the cancer was responding to treatment, I went on a ten-day mindfulness retreat at the Insight Meditation Center in Barre, Massachusetts. I felt I needed to practice, practice and practice some more to manage my anxiety about my upcoming CAT scan. I also needed a break and some time to replenish. Even though we were not supposed to do any writing I brought my journal along. Here are some excerpts.

6:30 am, Sunday, Early AM Meditation

This is the last time that we are instructed to use the breath as the prime vehicle of attention and I get it, finally! I experience being breathed (this means I'm relaxed and not trying to exert control over my breath). My attention is strong. As soon as I notice how good I'm doing I'm thinking again. This time it's about volition. What is under my control? Friday is my CAT scan and I want all my cancer to be gone. I fear it will not be. Should I tune into the universe and do Reiki on myself or imagine as I breathe that the cancer cells are seared, zapped, evaporated and then dissolved and released as I breathe out? I say to myself, "Just relax."

I return to my breath and notice:

In breath. Out breath.

What is skillful means?
How much should I actually do?
Can I trust myself to surrender to whatever happens?
Can I be assured that all that is needed is being done?

Next thought — This is it.
. . . .tightening in my chest
Thought. Am I using my time right?
Realization. I am thinking.
. . . .Back to my breath. Question dissolves.
Next thought.
"I'll create a workshop entitled
          THIS IS IT — VOLITION vs. SURRENDER
Does it matter?"
Next thought.
In-breath. Out-breath.
I can give myself suggestions, tune into the universe, heal, forget about it, whatever it is, and be breathed. I'm breathing anyway.
"Busy. Busy. Busy."

In breath. Out breath.

As I feel the wind brushing my face, as I sip my tea, I am aware of all the love in my life and I feel blessed. To be able to laugh — to kiss — to cry — to feel my knees aching from sitting on my cushion here in the meditation hall. How wonderful.

Not yet, please. If my time is soon I shall go in peace. But I want to grow old and beautiful with wrinkles around my eyes from laughing. I want to love many people and help heal their hearts. I want to bring joy to those who suffer, love to those who are afraid, peace to those who fear. I want to be breathing in and out, through boredom, wanting, anger and aversion, restlessness, doubt and fear for many more times.

Corrado Pensa, my meditation teacher, says these negative feelings are hindrances, cries for help.

Help! Help. Help me live as I breathe. Help me live as I walk and defecate and sleep. Help me love fully. Help!

CANCER — GO! DEATH — NOT YET!

Yesterday as I walked past a brook I thought how lovely it would be to sit under a tree and listen to the flowing stream smoothing out the rocks, bringing life to the pond and the animals that come; like the heron I saw yesterday at the pond by IMS.

NOT YET, PLEASE.

I want to walk holding David's hand and feel our bodies connected, our hearts entwined. I want to cook in our new kitchen and wash the floor and plant flowers indoors and out, paint pictures, dance and exercise, have people over and be free.

PLEASE — NOT YET.

Not yet time for breath to stop — thoughts to cease — curiosity to end or for this body that is mine to end — the mind to still . . . not yet, not yet.

BUT, the stream will flow on, the garden will still grow, the trees, heavy now with baby cones will propagate anew. . . . and Elana, will she continue to be?

We will see. We will see.

In the meantime
It is she who writes this ode
This plea . . . to continue . . . to be.

Friday evening

CAT SCAN FRIDAY
Now the birds are chirping
The chipmunks prance about
Looking for a nut,
A crumb.
Busy being alive.

The grass is green.
I am not ready to go.
Not yet.

The vegetable garden lush
With lettuce and peas,
Kale and beets,
Marigolds.

Death comes.
It is natural.
But.
Not now

Not yet, please.
The violets are just blooming.
Let my breath come and go many more times.

My heart opens wide
To sky that envelopes us here.

To each sunset,
Every step, each sight,
To eyes that smile,
As we pay attention and mindfully
Wake our sleepy selves.

Please,
Not yet.

Must I
Face death
To appreciate life?

Saturday, Tea Time

Ah, tea time, 5:30 p.m. Saturday. Retreat ending. I realize that at this moment I feel a little lost and incomplete. "This is it" keeps coming into my mind. And the song, "Racing with the clock" from the Pajama Game. I went for my CAT scan yesterday. It feels like it has taken me a long time to quiet down again after being away only an afternoon and evening.

The CAT scan showed enlarged nodes . . . again. I thought the cancer was gone . . . dissolved.

"Fight, fight, fight." I shall. I will. I do . . . but I am also tired.

As I munch my tea time snack, the chipmunks scamper by, one daring to go under my legs before it runs off. The pine trees are heavy with cones. There is something lovely and sweet about sitting, walking, breathing and eating with so many others also with the same intention to experience peace, to feel fulfillment and stillness. To be alive and awake.

A thunderstorm just blew by, dramatically clearing the air. I feel like running through the puddles in the wind like a little girl again, feeling the pleasure and wildness of the wind and the rain and the storm. Instead, I sit with the other adult children and observe — yes, Dad — with all my senses.

Later, standing under the portico of IMS, I breathe in the dampness and gaze up at the sky, now blue. One woman picks up branches from the path, downed by the storm; another, a younger one, sits on the steps, her long hair wet with rain. Watching. There is peace here and I feel protected, for a while, from the charge of life's "challenges." There's no need for money, no details of maintaining a household, a job, and a relationship. Only silence, teacher talks and yogi jobs . . . and my mind, seeing more clearly how everything changes.

And the winds come and the clouds go and the sun now beats strong.

How wonderful to feel this peace. This is what I hope to bring home with me.

GUIDED MEDITATION: AWARENESS OF THOUGHT

For this meditation, we will focus on thought and the process of thinking. This is an advanced practice and is best to do after there is a familiarity with meditation and the mind is steady.

TO BEGIN, ASSUME YOUR meditation position, one that supports your ability to concentrate and quiet. As with the other meditations, make sure that you will not be interrupted by phone calls or external demands. Remember, this is a time for you to *observe the workings of your mind without judgment.*

You can start by bringing your awareness to your breath. Allow your breath to anchor you to the present moment. You will also notice sound, sensation, and thought but let it be background as you focus on the process of breathing. Note what arises in your awareness but return to the breath.

When your attention is steady you can let the breath recede as your primary object of attention and open to thought as your focus. It is important to stay grounded in the present moment as you do this. When a thought enters your awareness, simply note it. If you like you can label it, such as: judgment, expectation, opinion, or worry (past or future). You can notice how one thought leads to another, and how easy it is to be swept away by thinking. Perhaps, as you give yourself permission to observe the thinking process, the mind will be quiet. Noticing this can precipitate a thought. Simply observe. If you find yourself being lost in thought, return to your breath or to sound, steady yourself in the present moment, and then return to the observation of thinking.

EXERCISE: PLEASANT VS. UNPLEASANT

If something is very painful or difficult it is natural to want to avoid it or push it away because it is unpleasant. Sometimes this is useful in order to be able to continue functioning and not be overwhelmed by "the problem," but if the problem doesn't really go away it can manifest itself in symptoms of stress mentally and physically. It can be helpful to keep a diary for a week and simply observe *without judging* what you experience as pleasant and unpleasant and jot down its effect on body and mind. Observe which is easiest to notice.

UNPLEASANT EVENTS DIARY

Be as specific as you can.	Sun	Mon	Tue	Wed	Thu	Fri	Sat
Describe the experience.							
Describe what you noticed in body.							
What moods, and feelings accompanied the event?							
What thoughts?							

Additional Reflections:

PLEASANT EVENTS DIARY

Be as specific as you can.	Sun	Mon	Tue	Wed	Thu	Fri	Sat
Describe the experience.							
Describe what you noticed in body.							
What moods, and feelings accompanied the event?							
What thoughts?							

Additional Reflections:

CONNECTION: WE'RE ALL IN THIS TOGETHER

Peace

When it comes
Is a surprise

To my mind
Trying so hard
To figure "it" out.

How much choice do I really have
As I walk the line between doing and being done?

Trust.

Relief will come.
If only I can

Smile.

Fresh from retreat, my awareness of grief and disappointment
was acute. I'd hoped that I'd be one of those miraculous patients
whose cancer just disappeared. Instead, I learned I'd need more
treatments of chemotherapy, and that a positive outcome was not
assured. In my journal I wrote:

I am afraid not to listen to the doctors but I really don't want more chemotherapy. I'm afraid that its effects will debilitate me permanently. I know it will increase my fatigue level.

On retreat, it had been easy to return to the present moment; all I had to do was sit, walk, eat, and do my yogi job. My thoughts came and went. Teaching nourished me, but I wondered if I was being present with all the concerns, longings, and pain that arose in class. How could I respond to the patients' comments about chronic pain or the muscle degeneration of muscular sclerosis or even chronic headaches? I was being worn down by chemotherapy. I wore bright scarves and looked cheerful and somewhat exotic, but my oomph faded easily. It was clear that patient and teacher were united in a common struggle to be well, even while tired or in pain.

In class, we could be honest and say, "This is hard work." In acknowledging the difficulty of this challenge *and not dwelling in it,* we cheered each other on and felt nourished. I felt as though my patients were my source of inspiration and I hoped I was theirs, but who knew for sure? In the class were a group of interns, observing. They were helpful in giving feedback, but they, too, needed attention. Class lasted two-and-a-half hours, as did the meeting with the interns after the class. By the end of the five hours I was exhausted, though stimulated.

Is equanimity the ability to tolerate my worry and grief and still feel joy and appreciation for what I do have?

With fresh eyes, I examined my life. What supported my well-being? Conversely, what threatened it? I looked around me. Our house, that I had once found charming, now felt tight and dark. I craved light and space. Was this under my control to change?

Visiting a friend who lived in a home that faced a small pond, I noticed a FOR SALE sign on another house on the street. It, too, faced the pond and there was a brook on the property and a large yard. The house looked comfortable and homey.

One Saturday, I convinced David to visit a realtor. I showed her the house and David reluctantly went with me for a viewing. He had no desire to move and was humoring me. In the house we saw the spacious living room and a dining area that looked out on the pond. Upstairs, through a room that had been converted to a study, we stepped outside onto a concrete roof covering the patio below. The cold, crisp air of a clear winter night tingled on my skin as we looked out onto the yard, illuminated by moon and spotlights. The white snow seemed to stretch forever, across the pond and beyond. Ash and birch trees stood silently beautiful in the yard, their branches cushioned by snow. We could hear the sounds of night and see the stars and the ring of snow-covered fir trees lining the side of the property. It transported us far from Worcester and worries. David could imagine a hot tub there. I stopped thinking.

The house itself was interesting, with a curved art deco iron-railed staircase and enough rooms for David and me to have our own studies. There were large windows facing the outside and it was light and airy. I could imagine living in the house and having room for an office and mini-retreats. It felt welcoming and hospitable, a healing, meditative environment. Using money we had inherited from my father when he died, we decided to take the plunge and buy.

"Life is what it's all about," said Pablo Neruda. "I want no truck with death."

We moved in September, the day after my next-to-last chemotherapy treatment. I was so excited I stayed up until two or three in the morning, sitting on the floor, surrounded by boxes and paper. I unpacked boxes as if I were possessed. I unwrapped my mother's crystal and placed it in the cabinet from my parents' house that now lined my dining room wall. I hung pictures and an old framed photo of my great-grandmother that I placed next to a brass mask we had brought back from a trip to India and a non-working wooden barometer that had hung on my parents' living room wall. I took the hats my father had collected and hung them on the coat rack in the hall. I unwrapped our dishes and silverware so we could eat and have breakfast at home the next day. As I decorated the walls and filled the cabinets, my mind quieted. I was home.

I had my final chemotherapy treatment as the leaves were turning color. Six months passed. I went for my check-up and had another

CAT scan. Once again, it was discovered that the cancer was growing. By now it was spring and the forsythia was just beginning to bud.

I was in the middle of a teaching cycle. We were in the section on stress, a time in class when people are beginning to notice more acutely how their own reactions to events intensify the stress in their lives. It is often a time of doubt and discouragement, the dark before the light, when people need an extra boost of trust and faith that meditating and becoming more aware will help them cope and feel better. The class keeps a diary of stressors, noting what precipitates a stress reaction and the thoughts, sensations, feelings and actions that accompany it. This is observed *without judgment.*

My reaction to my own news was one of disbelief and shock. My life had just begun to return to normalcy and I was finally finding that I had more energy. I had been going regularly for acupuncture and taking Chinese herbs. I was exercising and meditating. I had hoped to prevent a recurrence. I didn't want my life to be interrupted. Now I understood why it was so hard for the members of my class to have the endurance to stay with their thoughts and feelings when they experienced stress. It was unpleasant.

I had been told that the longer I was in remission, the better were my chances of survival. This recurrence so soon meant a poorer prognosis. Tests indicated that the cancer was becoming more virulent and moving more toward an intermediate grade. This meant it was growing more rapidly. The tumors in my neck were larger and I had others of a more aggressive type in the pelvic area. I would not have long to live unless I took some drastic action.

Since I had already received the maximum number of standard chemotherapy treatments, eight, my only hope for long-term survival would be an autologous peripheral stem cell transplant. This is a serious procedure involving heavy doses of chemotherapy that destroys good cells as well as cancerous ones. For this reason, stem cells, the cells produced in the marrow that manufacture the white and red blood cells necessary for health, are harvested. To do this, I'd be hooked up to a special machine that would harvest the cells from a vein in my arm. They are then stored and transplanted into the vein after the chemotherapy has wiped out all the cells in the marrow.

This is called day zero, a time when the risk of infection is very high. I'd be hospitalized for at least three weeks, possibly more.

It would take a minimum of six months for my immune system to recover after hospitalization. To protect myself during this time, I wouldn't be able to enter public places or be inside with more than one or two people. I could eat no uncooked fruits or vegetables and my residence would have to be as germ-free as possible. That meant applying bleach to kitchen counters, putting away plants, and having no flowers in the house. I'd even have to empty the fountain in my living room. Any receptacles that could harbor harmful bacteria or fungi had to be eliminated. It was also suggested that we get rid of our dog, which I decided I would not do.

My overwhelming feeling is that of grief . . . I also notice fear and feel myself girding up to have the strength for more battle. My challenge is to stay in the present moment . . . I have had to ask myself whether the risk and hardship I will experience is worth the effort. Can I accept the outcome of my decision, whatever it will be? If I choose to have the transplant can I accept any negative consequences that arise? If I choose to do nothing will I be at peace knowing there was an alternative?

I felt good, but I feared being sick again. I dreaded more treatment, but I also wanted to be alive as long as feasibly possible. I realized it wasn't only my life I needed to consider, but also my husband's. He didn't want to lose me. This made it very hard to say, "No, I won't have a transplant. I'll take my chances."

I consulted my Chinese physician, who was a consultant to the National Institute of Health. He, and his teacher, after checking my pulse and examining me, urged me to have the transplant. "The cancer" they said, "is growing too fast for herbs to stop it now."

Once I decided to have the procedure, there were still other decisions to be made. I needed to choose which hospital, which doctors, which regimen, all of them slightly different and very confusing to sort out. More than ever, meditation helped me by bringing relief and stillness, if not instant clarity, to my choices. I was on new ground. Researchers were still investigating what worked and what did not. Ultimately, I opted for proximity to home and an environment I trusted, the University of Massachusetts Medical

School where I worked and had friends. The doctor, Dr. Pam Becker, treated me with respect and I could talk to her. The transplant unit was new and all its personnel had been hand-picked. I felt secure that I'd get excellent care.

Being able to finish teaching my stress reduction class was now impossible and the yoke of responsibility weighed heavy on me. I hoped that I could teach one or two more classes before I'd have to go into the hospital for my first round of chemotherapy. It was a delicate time in class and I wanted to be able to guide us through "Stress and our reaction to it." I didn't like admitting that I was upset and having to exert all my energy to maintain my equilibrium.

I remember sitting down at the next week's teachers' meeting, sighing deeply, and saying, "If I didn't have to, I wouldn't teach tomorrow."

All of the teachers looked at me and said, "You don't have to. We'll help you."

I sat there, stunned. It never occurred to me I could stop teaching.

In-breath, out-breath.

I knew I was upset and tired, but until that moment I hadn't realized how tightly I had been holding on to my identity as a teacher, or how forbidden it was for me to admit vulnerability. It felt like shirking responsibility.

Not teaching meant admitting that I was very sick with a life-threatening disease that required drastic, invasive measures for survival. It meant acknowledging that I was tired and scared and that my energy was being zapped by fear and grief and anticipatory worries. It meant recognizing that chemotherapy would weaken me and that I'd need hospitalization and a six-month recuperation period . . . if I survived the procedure. It was too much to fully grasp consciously, but internally it rang true: I shouldn't teach.

I wanted to be a model for my class, but teaching regardless of circumstances was false. The kindness and compassion of my friends, my colleagues, helped me see the truth of my situation. They didn't say, "You're bad. How could you stop now in the middle of the cycle?"

I was saying that to myself. My dear colleagues were loving and concerned. It was a transformative moment.

Acknowledging the severity of the problem and addressing my diagnosis head on by NOT teaching and using my time for self-care was the right course of action. Denying that my life had changed, or that my tasks were now different, was not helpful.

AND I DIDN'T LIKE IT.

Slowly, it sunk in, I didn't have to like it, I simply had to respond to the truth, and then I could relax and do what *really* needed to be done: I had to prepare myself, mentally and physically, for transplant.

The compassion and understanding behind the words "you don't have to . . . we'll help you," penetrated my grief and woke me up. I no longer felt that I had to hold and support the twenty-two people in my class. As my perspective shifted, the heaviness I had been feeling lifted.

"We'll help you."

My colleagues saw clearly. They heard me, saw me, and recognized my deep need to maintain my pride and take care of myself. Without judging or pitying me, they helped me let go. I didn't have to teach. What a relief. They respected the fatigue of my spirit, as well as my body, more than I did.

Simply notice how you react without judging it.
Once you are aware, you have choices and can do what is needed.

My "shoulds" and "ought to's" dissolved, freeing me from the box I hadn't known I had created.

As I took in, "You don't have to; we'll help you," struggle ceased. A deep sense of gratitude arose and on a very deep level I now knew that the love and sense of connection I felt with others could not be severed even though they were "healthy" and I had cancer. We were all in this together.

Later on, they joked about the outfit I wore to the meeting, a beige suit I had just bought on sale with vertical stripes.

"You usually dress so elegantly," said Florence.

"You look like a prisoner," Saki added.

That was how I had felt when I entered the room. Now I could give it away to Goodwill Industries.

With sadness and relief, it was decided that my colleague, Ferris Urbanowski, would come to my next class with me. I would tell the class what happened and pass the reins to her. She'd teach this class and the next and then Florence Meyer would teach the final two classes. I would remain as long as I could, but as "patient."

The next day, Ferris and I went to class together. As the class members took their seats along the walls of the room, we placed ourselves in the center. I began with a meditation:

> *Letting go of everything but this moment,*
> *allow yourself to leave behind work*
> *and the thoughts of the day that has passed,*
> *or the evening to come.*
> *Simply follow your breath.*
> *As you breathe in, bring your attention fully to the in-breath*
> *and as you breathe out bring it fully to the out-breath,*
> *allowing it to be as it is*
> *without trying to change it in any way.*

We sat for a few minutes so that everyone could settle in and then I rang the bells, looked around the room at the people present, took a deep breath, and introduced Ferris.

"Ferris is a good friend and a wonderful teacher. She will be taking over the class. I've just learned that the lymphoma I've had has returned and I will need more chemotherapy and some hospitalization."

Everyone, including the interns observing and participating in the class, was very quiet, looking at me intently.

"I would like to stay in class with you, but now it will be as a patient. Ferris, and then Florence Meyer, will continue on as the teachers."

I stood up, moved from the center of the room to an empty chair along the side and sat down. Ferris waited a moment or two and asked, "What is it that people are experiencing now?"

Sitting back in my chair along the wall, I was filled with emotion, my breathing fast, my throat constricted. I recall listening intently to what people said, but can only remember the seriousness of tone and the heaviness of feeling in my chest and in the room. When it was my turn, it was hard to speak. Never before had I felt it was permissible to acknowledge weakness and be vulnerable in public without feeling that it was shameful or bad.

Teary-eyed, I shifted position and said, "I've never before been able to state what I needed and have it received and fulfilled as wholeheartedly and fully as now. I feel very thankful and blessed. I thank everyone here."

And led by Ferris, we moved on to discuss our homework and our reactions to stress.

SUPPORTS: AN EXERCISE IN AWARENESS

External as well as internal factors can support your well-being. It can be useful to take some time to note what *currently* in your life helps you be well and encourages creativity and hope. There are often simple things which we take for granted that can make a difference in how we feel. For example, I find I respond to light and sunny days. I notice that sitting in a room that is well lit and painted in a cheerful color can uplift my spirit. I find that dressing in bright colors can also improve my mood. I love the feel of the water on my skin when I take a shower. I respond positively to a smile.

GET INTO A COMFORTABLE position and, allowing your body and mind to relax, take a few moments and ask yourself the question, *What supports my well-being?*

Let your mind go through your day(s) and take note of what helped quiet or comfort you or made you smile. You may then jot down what comes to mind and continue to pay attention as you move through your activities, adding to your list as you notice the supports already in place in your relationships, work and environment.

Simply note what comes to mind, letting go of any judging thoughts or self-criticism for what is not yet in place. If you like, you can keep a daily diary noting the feelings, thoughts and sensations that arise that facilitate well-being and ease of living.

Remember, the small stuff is important. The more you can bring into awareness moments that carry peace and joy, the happier you can be.

WHAT SUPPORTS ME IN MY LIFE

A Daily Record

	Sun	Mon	Tue	Wed	Thu	Fri	Sat
Home							
Leisure							
People							
Work							

Pay attention to your environment, relationships, use of time and the choices you are making that support your health.

After you've completed this exercise, you might want to take the time to jot down what DOESN'T support your well-being yet is under your control to change. Next to it, write down what YOU CAN incorporate in your life to enhance your well-being and COMMIT YOURSELF to an action plan and timetable. You may change this as you go along, but it is useful to write it down to help you get started implementing these plans.

Be realistic as you do this evaluation. Create a plan with steps that you can implement NOW and be successful in accomplishing. One step builds on another. You might want to take your calendar and your appointment book and schedule in time for this plan so it becomes a part of your day. If there are attitudinal changes you'd like to make, write them down, create a slogan for yourself and place it where you can see it and be inspired to incorporate them in your life.

Roots

Awesome. Frightening.
Being
in the
Unknown.

Growing roots.

Roots of Courage,
Roots of Strength,
Roots of Determination,
Affirmation.

Roots
Pushing Down,
Roots,
Pushing through.

Beat the weeds back
Push, strain, sweat.

Roots
Pushing through the soil.
Roots.

Roots of desire
Roots of hope
Seeking,
Groping,
for
Elements
that
Sustain life.

I stopped teaching, but I refused to give up my summer vacation, three weeks at the beach. Bekka, my eleven-year-old niece, would be visiting us for one of those weeks and we were really looking forward to time away and time with her. My veins, scarred from eight previous treatments, could not withstand a new assault of chemo-therapy

without a tube, a catheter that gave direct access to an artery. I elected
to have a porta-catheter planted under my skin, rather than an external
one, so I could go swimming and not be encumbered with the special
care an external one would require. Four days after it was implanted,
when the area around it was still swollen, I went into the hospital for
four days of chemotherapy. From there, I planned to go directly to
the beach.

In the hospital by my bed was my journal, colored pencils, and
some books. This was the first time I had been hospitalized and I
didn't like it.

*Karate Chop to Cancer, Chemo and porta-catheters, hospitals,
    Johnnies, and the indignity of being . . . A PATIENT!*

"You're such a good sport," they said.

"I wouldn't have let them do that to me," said the well-meaning
Sister of Mercy.

"Was there a choice?" I asked.

The attempt to access my porta-catheter required 14 pricks with
a large needle. The whole process brought tears to my eyes and I
didn't have the oomph to tell the staff to stop. I wish I had been less
stoic, less successful at breathing into the pain and enduring it quietly.
The helpless feeling that comes over me is worse than physical pain.
At those times I become too good a patient, too worn out to make
the effort to assert myself. It didn't even occur to me that I have the
power to tell the staff to cease what they're doing, that there are
alternatives.

*I don't know what will be next. Will it be more pain, more surgery,
help or hurt? And sometimes the two go together. Ah. More challenge!*

*My room is in a Catholic hospital. A crucifix arrests my attention.
I'm finding it troublesome to look at it. I feel nailed to a cross. I'm not
freely able to move and I have a needle and tubing sticking out from my
chest through which toxins are entering.*

When my colleague, Rafaella, who is also a Lutheran minister,
was visiting me, I said, "Rafaela, how is this crucifix inspiring?"

"He's suffering for you," she said, "taking on your pain so you
can heal."

I didn't understand. I am Jewish, not of this tradition and I couldn't get beyond the pain. I started wondering about all my years as a therapist. Did I take on the pain of others and get lost in it? Had I been able to release it or had it stuck to me? Is this why I had cancer?

Back to the here and now.

"Can you tell me more about transcending pain?" I asked Rafella.

"Yes. On Good Friday I am grieved, sad, and in pain. On Easter I am filled with joy. They go together."

Compassionately, she took the carving of a suffering Christ off the wall and placed it gently in another place. It came down easily. Helping me understand was healing. I felt she embodied the crucifix's meaning.

Being a patient thrust me into a new position. I wanted to convert my experience into guidelines for teaching my classes. My colleague, Fernando, was beginning teaching in the stress reduction program and had recently visited me. His visit sparked me to write:

NOTES TO TEACHERS

Recently, I was speaking to Fernando and found myself naming three guidelines for teaching:

1) Really be with each person in the class.
2) Focus on Practice-Practice-Practice.
3) Do not be afraid to go to the heart of the matter.

I'll begin with the third point. Fernando and I were talking about the art of being direct and penetrating delusion. He was saying how he didn't want to hurt or offend anyone. This brought to mind my experience in the hospital. A porta-catheter had been inserted in my chest to allow easy access to my veins for the drawing of blood and the infusion of chemo. It was under my skin so I could go swimming and easily shower and bath and be free of having to care for it. The first time it had to be accessed so that I could receive chemotherapy, the nurse couldn't get into it. She stuck me once, twice and then said she couldn't do it. I was passed to the oncology nurse. She too felt my chest, looked at my suture where the catheter had been inserted, and taking out the special needle designed to access this port, a needle thick and long, again punctured my skin without success of entry.

This went on throughout the day. No one wanted to hurt me. The surgeon who had done the implant was called. "Go through the suture," he said. Yet everyone was reluctant to do so; they didn't want to cause me pain. All afternoon I continued to be passed from surgical resident to nurse. Finally, after ten attempts I ended up in radiology. Under the fluoroscope, the port could be clearly seen but once again, the needle was inserted and no blood could be drawn. Finally, after three more attempts, one of the technicians took the plunge, went straight through the suture and deep down into the skin. Success!

The desire not to hurt me had made ineffective the attempts to help me and literally prolonged what I had to endure. So now I instruct others, "Be precise, go to the point directly, penetrate as deep as needed. The fear of hurting someone needs to be respected but be wise, it can also serve to prolong suffering."

Bekka arrived from California on my last day in the hospital. It must have been difficult for her to see me as I was, bald and hooked up to tubes. She brought me some terrific stick-um tattoos of ice cream cones to decorate my bald head, helped me wet and put them on and then wrote in my journal:

> *To let go,*
> *To leave behind.*
> *NO.*
> *NEVER!*
>
> *To plunge.*
> *To close your eyes forever.*
> *NO!*
>
> *I refuse.*
> *I will fight.*
> *Forever.*
> *I will not let go.*
> — Bekka Rosenbaum, age 11, 8/7/96

Thank you, Bekka. I won't let go, either. I won't give up or surrender to depression, hatred and self-pity. This is under my control.

EXERCISE: GOING TO THE HEART OF THE MATTER

TAKE YOUR MEDITATION position. Allow your mind to settle, carving space and time for yourself to quiet and come into the present moment, letting everything go but your focus of attention, be it breath or the passing flow of sound, thoughts, feelings or sensations. When you feel the mind to be steady and solidly grounded in the present moment, you can ask yourself to bring to mind a situation that troubles you.

Simply notice what arises, being aware of thoughts, feelings and sensations but continuing to use your breath as an anchor so that you don't get swept away into the experience. If it's helpful, you can imagine yourself sitting in a movie in a comfortable seat and watching the show as if it were on the screen. *Simply observe without judging.* Put in as many details as possible. Where does the scene take place? When? With whom? Does it happen often or only at special times or in certain circumstances? Can you identify the triggers? Notice your place in the situation. What is your body position? What sensations are you feeling? Do you speak? If so, are you "making nice" and trying to placate, or might you over-react and be aggressive? What emotions do you notice?

As you do this, remember to continue to feel the movement of breath. You can stop at any time and continue with the sensation of breathing to steady yourself and be able to witness the scene without reacting. When you are again calm and quiet, return to the event.

As the scene becomes clear to you, notice if there is something that you could say or do to alter your response or affect the outcome of this situation. Mentally be assertive respectfully but firmly stating what you want or need. Take a moment and jot down the statement and then rehearse it in your mind. Then try it out verbally, noting your tone of voice, phrasing and body position. If you like you can do this in front of a mirror or into a tape recorder. Notice again thoughts, feelings and sensations as you mentally explore different scenarios.

Be as authentic in your response as possible. You can repeatedly ask yourself, *"What is the truth of this situation? Am I penetrating to the heart of the matter? What choices do I have?"*

Remember, this is for you. You have choices, and you can choose NOT to do anything. The goal is to achieve self-respect and a sense of internal freedom and peace.

ROOTS: A GUIDED MEDITATION

It has become a habit of mine to look out the window. I find myself doing it as punctuation between thoughts. It takes me out of myself to another dimension. By the window where I sit are some fir trees. I observe them standing straight and tall, and silent. I notice when they are bowed down, laden with snow. I see them moving with the wind, bending and straightening. The branches jut out, perpendicular to the trunk. I observe the needles: tiny and precise, connected to branches that attach to other branches, extending out laterally to receive the sun.

The birch trees also visible are beautiful, graceful and slender. They are stark now and leafless on this winter day, waiting for spring thaw and a bird to nest in the hollow of its trunk. In spring and summer, the leaves reach up into the brightness of sky and sun.

When I painted a mural on my bedroom walls the sky was blue and serenity greeted me when I woke up. The scene had depth, variety, and color. It lived with me not only on the walls of my room but in my imagination.

IF YOU LIKE, YOU CAN allow yourself to get into your meditation position, sitting upright with dignity and in comfort or lying down with arms alongside your body. Allow your eyes to close. Take a few moments to ground yourself by opening to sound, letting it come to you as you rest here in the now of this moment.

You can let go of everything but listening. Hear sound as it comes and goes, and notice its qualities such as tone, loudness, and softness. Doing nothing, but letting yourself receive what comes within your hearing.

As your mind steadies, you may notice the subtle movement of your body as you breathe. If you like, you can let your attention rest on your breath, noticing where it is most vivid for you. Sensations, thoughts and feelings may enter your awareness and you can note them as background as you continue feeling the rhythm of your breath and listening to sounds. Notice how you are breathing in and breathing out. Let the breath be your anchor, helping you ride the waves of thought, feelings and bodily sensations.

And once you feel quiet you can, if you like, let yourself imagine being a tree. Notice what type it is. What season of the year is it? How does this affect it? Let the image or feel of a tree come to you and notice what connects most easily to your spirit.

You can bring awareness to the size of its trunk, its bark, its shape, height and girth, noticing where it stands, noticing its relationship to its environment, the ground and the sky. Is it a mature tree or a sapling? You can experiment with both.

Notice and breathe with the tree as it enters into your awareness either visually or as a felt sense, strong and steady, reaching out to the elements that sustain life. You can imagine the tree growing tall and strong, vital and healthy, venerable and wise as it puts forth branches and leaves, and grows new sprouts from its root system. Notice how the branches reach out to touch the sun. Let yourself feel the air and the space around the tree, above and below and all around, that give it room to breathe and be well.

And in your mind's eye, notice the extensive root system that nourishes and supports the tree. If you like you can imagine the roots going deep, deep down and spreading out laterally through the earth to receive moisture and nutrients. Perhaps you can see the tree covered with snow or bright with new spring foliage. And you can imagine it standing through all conditions as it moves with the wind and the weather, mild and warm, cold and dark, windy and clear, stormy or calm.

The tree stays rooted to the ground, pushing down new roots to support it through its life, day by day, hour by hour, moment by moment. You too can be flexible and strong, supported like the tree, as you move through the conditions of your life. Each breath anchors the roots of your tree firmly into the ground — to help you find what is nourishing so you may flourish.

Each time you return to your breath, each time you come back to the present moment, you can imagine your roots becoming stronger and keeping you upright as you move through seasons and climate, braving the elements of the mind, and your own wants and desires, disappointments and losses.

Take all the time you need to do this meditation. You may even choose to do it accompanied by music. When you feel that your image (or sense) of a tree, roots and branches is complete, notice its effect on your breath, your thoughts and your body. Then when you are ready, gently open your eyes and slowly move into an upright position and begin to draw the image that came to you. Remember to be free of judgment and let the tree and its root system evolve. It is a work in progress. Give yourself all the time, space, and rest you need to be able to flourish. If you like, imagine your tree connected to other trees, your root system intermingled with theirs, together standing strong and harmoniously.

If you like, you can name your tree, letting its name and its sound represent your strength, giving you hope, wisdom and freedom.

THE HEALING CEREMONY

The doctors were in charge when it came to my physical preparation for transplant, but my psychic preparation was under my own care. I had read studies indicating that prayer made a difference in a person's healing so I put aside false humility and called everyone who had been important in my life, whose telephone number I still had, including my ex-husband in Seattle, and asked them to pray for me. I also decided to have a healing ceremony before I entered the hospital for the transplant. I invited relatives, good friends, neighbors and all the staff at the Stress Reduction Clinic, as well as a favorite meditation teacher of mine.

It was the middle of September and the period between the Jewish New Year, Rosh Hashanah, and Yom Kippur. These ten days are days of reflection during which a person reviews his or her conduct for the past year and asks forgiveness for sins and transgressions between man and God and man and man. This includes speech as well as actions. This is a serious and holy time during which tradition says it is decided who shall live and who shall die. Each day a *shofar*, a ram's horn, is blown; its sound saying, "Wake up! Wake up! Listen! Hear! Open to the One."

On a Sunday afternoon, people gathered at the house. After all had arrived and greeted each other, we all moved outside onto the lawn in our backyard. Our friend, Alan Harris, blew the shofar to begin the ceremony. I was wearing my volcano dress, a fiery orange/ red silk caftan I had purchased in Hawaii a few years before. I had a bright colored scarf and a band around my head to keep it on. As we all sat down in a circle, I took off the scarf and sat bareheaded among all my friends.

We sat in silence and then Ellen Wingard blessed me with a Celtic prayer.

> *May the nourishment of the earth be yours.*
> *May the clarity of light be yours.*
> *May the fluency of ocean be yours.*
> *May the blessings that come from all who love*
> *you fill you and infuse you with healing.*
>
> *May the protection of ancestors be yours.*
> *May a slow wind of love surround you and fill*
> *you to mind your life in each minute.*

And I added, "And all that I receive, may it also be yours and fill you with blessings."

Again we sat in silence and then Melissa Blacker opened the bag of instruments she had brought and another friend his collection of drums to use for the ceremony.

"We can dance, we can sing, we can stomp and make a lot of noise," Melissa informed us.

"You can use your body to make sounds, use your hands, your feet. Listen to yourself and your wishes for Elana . . . from the silence, listen to everybody. Close your eyes and listen, and when you are ready, making sounds and sending it into Elana. And Elana sending it back into you."

As dusk began to fall, the drumming began, a strong steady rhythm that brought me to my feet. I walked around the circle, palms clasped together, moving my body up and down to the beat of the drums, in supplication and joy, bending, moving, swaying to the sounds of mariachis and sticks, a rain tube and voices. Around and around I went, moving slowly and solemnly acknowledging everyone in the circle, connecting to the earth and the sky and the rhythm. When I was finished, David rose and stomped into the center of the circle, chanting, "Go cancer, go. Stomp it out. Out with cancer. Out of her body . . . Completely."

My throat constricted. It was so powerful and moving to hear the force of his cry, the depth of his caring, his fear, and his desire. The drums continued to beat out.

"Go cancer, go."

David returned to the circle. Ned brought a candle into the center. The drumming went on. It was suggested that there be a hands-on healing for all who wished to do so and I was brought into the middle of the circle. People began chanting, "OMM."

The tones were deep and low and continuous. It reminded me of a Gregorian chant. And then we chanted, "*Shalom; Peace.*"

"Let's bring David into the circle."

He joined me as people continued to chant and sing. Someone lit a torch and as we began to sing a Hebrew song, *He Nay Mah Tov.* (Here we are together in friendship. It is good and filled with joy.) We went back to our places and Ned handed out votive candles glued onto round wooden floats he had made. I stood with a torch and everyone rose with their lit candles and walked toward the brook, the light illuminating the dark. One by one, each person bent down and placed his or her candle in the water, flames of light floating gently on the water as we stood singing, "*We shall overcome. We shall overcome. We are not afraid. Deep in my heart, I do believe, we shall overcome someday.*"

We continued singing as we watched the circles of light move slowly into the pond,

"*Oh, we delight in the light of the river flowing so gently to the strength of the sea. We take delight in the love that is flowing just like a river in the love that's among us.*"

We went on to "*We got the whole world in our hands,*" and "*Joshua fought the battle of Jericho, Jericho, and the walls came tumbling down.*"

Darkness had fallen and only the candles illuminated the dark. We returned to the house and Nerina, who was a native of Australia and had studied with the aborigines, took a hair from her head and asked each person present to add onto it, spinning it together, and with it place their prayer and intention for me. She explained this was an aborigine-healing amulet that the person to be healed wore as a pin or bracelet. Since everything on the transplant unit needed to be sterile, I could take mine and place it in a baggy, which I later did. I carried it with me when I entered the hospital a few days later.

Blessed, I now felt prepared for the rigors of hospitalization and stem cell transplant.

EXERCISE: A HEALING CEREMONY

Sometimes we have to go outside our usual routine and mode of being in order to acknowledge a major shift or mark a significant occasion in our lives. It is very useful to mark an important event and create a ritual to honor it. Traditionally, this is done in a community and often a religious setting. However, it can also be a personal ritual, a time to stop, reflect, and commemorate the occasion. This can be done in a time of crisis or joy.

Is there any ritual you would like to create? If so, would this be one for yourself, or would you like to include others? What would be meaningful for you? Is there any particular music you would like to use? Singing? What do you find inspirational? Do you have favorite poems or readings? Are there any special prayers or religious ceremonies that you would like to incorporate in your ritual? Who would you like to invite to share it with you? Do you want to choose someone to lead it or do it yourself?

Let your mind imagine different possibilities, asking yourself how they might nourish and support you? You can be free to be creative or repeat a familiar custom. Enjoy, appreciate, and allow yourself to receive. This will give to others, as well as to yourself.

TRANSPLANT

I knew my body would be assaulted by chemotherapy during my transplant, but I was determined to keep my spirit hardy. I wasn't afraid of being isolated; after all, hadn't I practiced being solitary on retreats? I was comfortable with quiet and the idea of staying in a sealed room (to protect me from infection) didn't bother me, although it was important for my spirit to have windows and light. Fortunately, the corner room in the hospital, with two large windows, was available. The bed in it faced the west, with a beautiful view of the historic state hospital that stood like a castle high on a hillside surrounded by greenery.

The transplant unit was on the eighth floor, the top floor of the hospital. If I looked diagonally across and down from my room, I could see the Stress Reduction Clinic's classroom. I was told later that everyone in the classes used to look up at my window and send me Metta, wishing me to be safe and protected, happy, healthy and at ease.

The room itself was bare, except for a stationary bike on one end, an outlet for a PC, and high tech equipment for my infusions of chemotherapy and stem cells. There was also a small surveillance camera mounted on the ceiling and pointed at the bed. Nearby a TV/VCR was bolted to the wall.

I had read that it was very important to make the environment comfortable and supportive of healing, so I arrived on the unit wheeling a cart borrowed from pediatrics loaded with "stuff." It included a large framed poster, *The Fauve Landscape*, that my father had given me years ago, a picture of brightly colored boats moored by the promenade of a fishing village in southern France. It was bright and cheerful. I put it on the floor across from the bed where I could see it. It was painted in vivid blues and greens, oranges and gold, and seemed to shout, "Live, enjoy!" Looking at it, I could feel the verve and life of the scene, a counterbalance to the sterility of the room.

I also brought along the colored pencils I had carried with me to chemotherapy sessions, waiting rooms and my preparatory hospitalization. I had a selection of CDs, earphones, my computer, books, (inspirational ones on meditation, as well as mysteries and science fiction), cards, as well as videos of musicals that a friend had collected and given me to watch. In addition, I had the woven hair of all of my friends from the healing ceremony. I don't think the nurses or doctors had ever seen anything like this.

My perspective was, "I'll get through this." I did not think about death. I focused on being in the moment. Again and again, I remember saying to myself, "This is it. This is what is happening. This moment counts as much as the moments when I am physically healthy and active."

I knew I had to put aside my doubts and stay present with my experience in order to get through it. Now I understood the importance of staying put on one's cushion and deepening the ability to be steady, simply observing the show of mind states, feelings and bodily sensations coming and going. I hoped the experience wouldn't be too bad and I had faith that I'd survive.

"Everything passes," I told myself. "This, too, shall pass." And it was wonderfully helpful to gaze out at the sky. It seemed so big and endless and I so small. It helped put my pain and my concerns in perspective.

I only have selected memories of my time on the unit: the warmth and care of the nurses; David's visits, often spent reading to me; the joy of sucking on an orange popsicle, its cold soothing the sores that lined the inside of my mouth and prevented me from speaking or eating. I remember the warmth and care of people rather than the pain. I remember thinking that even if I were to die, life would continue, babies would be born, children would still laugh and seasons would arrive and go. It was reassuring to hear the sounds of children below my window and outside in the corridor and enjoy the spontaneity of their voices.

With the exception of the first and last couple of days, I was too sick to read, listen to music, or watch TV. My concentration was very short. I spent much of my time looking out the window, finding solace in the sky, watching it change color and observing the clouds. It was absorbing to watch the different formations and watch them float away. I insisted on keeping the blinds up in the room. The sunlight gave hope and its vastness soothed me.

This was especially important when I had pneumonia. Only now, as I write, can I begin to comprehend the fragility of my life during that period. Dr. Becker told me that never in her experience had she seen a person who was as seriously ill as I was, breathing with such difficulty, and receiving the maximum amount of oxygen possible, through a tube in my nose and a mask over my mouth, yet able to hold on without going on a respirator. I believe that is when I had David read me *The Little Engine that Could.*

"You're strong," Dr. Becker said. "A real stoic."

During this time I was hooked up to machines, dependent on oxygen for breath; I could not struggle. I didn't have the energy. It didn't make sense. All of heart, mind, body, will and me were directed toward survival. I remember Kamala Masters, a meditation teacher, and Franz Moeckl, who taught Qi Gong, coming to the room. I had studied with each of them. When they came, I couldn't talk. My mouth was filled with sores from the chemotherapy. My face was covered with an oxygen mask. The nurses and doctors were fearful that I might not survive.

I remember them entering the room, gazing at me, recognizing my stillness and simply sitting down. It seemed they brought peace with them. They were not afraid. They felt no need to talk to me, cheer me up, or give me anything material. Instead, they sat and meditated. Kamala tells me, now, that she repeated Metta again and again, sending me wishes of love, of health, of safety from harm and of ease of being. Even without words, I felt these wishes and was able to go to sleep. I surrendered. I felt held. I knew I was safe. All was well. Surrender brought peace and with it came all the freedom I ever wished to have.

Later, when I was well, that memory inspired me to return to the transplant unit and sit with others, to give to them what had been so freely given to me. But back then I had no room for thought, or even fight. I believe that I survived because I surrendered and let myself sink deep down into the quiet space I felt as I looked out at the sky. Breath by breath, I let myself be breathed. I sunk deeper down into the bed, into each slow, labored breath, and relaxed.

David came every day and sat on my bed, holding my hand in his gloved one. (Visitors had to wash their hands and don latex gloves and wear a mask over their noses and mouths.) He read aloud a chapter a day from *Kitchen Table Wisdom* by Rachel Naomi Remen. My friend, Elizabeth Wheeler, a psychologist in behavioral medicine, did hypnosis with me to help me imagine myself becoming stronger and recovering. I appreciated each person who prayed for me and sent me love. Like my father, each morning I felt lucky to be able to say, "I'm here."

Once, in the middle of the night, a new nurse woke me up to give me medication. I felt her apprehension as she tended to me. Her fear of my dying on her shift was contagious and suddenly I felt scared and became anxious. The darkness outside reflected the feeling inside. I repeated Metta to myself as I followed my breath. Eventually, it passed and I slept.

When the oxygen mask came off, I was very weak. It was a major effort to be able to move from the bed to my commode. When I was able to go to the bathroom, it was a thrill, but difficult. To walk down the corridor with my robe, mask, and IV pole, I needed assistance. I felt like a "big girl" when I could wash my own face and sponge myself off. Diane, my nurse, tells me I loved sitting in the warmth of the sitz bath, which she made for me.

Towards the end of my stay, one of the orderlies learned that my counts (blood cells) were up. As a special treat, she wheeled me outside. I remember the wonder of moving from the confines of my small, air-filtered room, through the hospital corridors and out the lobby door into the air. I felt liberated. I sat in my wheelchair and looked about. I marveled at the leaves now filled with color. I smelled the grass and the leaves. I experienced the sounds of activity and the wind brushing my face. I felt the warm moisture of air touching my bald head. It felt like heaven.

I was awestruck. Appreciation of life filled me with gratitude and wonder. Back on the unit, the doctors and nurses were impressed by my willpower and my equanimity. To me, what I had done was effortless and natural. I had simply relaxed. I felt there had been no other choice. As I became stronger, I wrote in my journal:

October 23

It is now 5:45 am. I haven't been able to sleep so I decided it was a perfect time to pick up my mail, which has been in cyberspace while I was too sick to turn on the computer. The teachers at the clinic are giving me a present of a foot massage this morning and I am excited. I'm also really ready to go home but I can't yet. I'm a little scared about what it will be like. I am being slowly weaned off of IV's. My prayer for each day is that nothing eventful happens. I would love a steady recovery without any surprises.

My eyes are lidded right now but I don't want to close them. There just seems to be so much feeling that I am holding: sadness, joy, grief, awe and fatigue. I have never come so close to death and I pray that David and I will be able to have many years together. To be able to breathe, to BE AWAKE, TO HAVE SOME ENERGY. *Consciousness is a miracle.*

I am tired . . . it is hard to concentrate. I look forward to my Cream of Wheat *for breakfast and* I WANT HOT CHOCOLATE WITH IT. **WANT.** IT'S GOOD TO WANT AGAIN! *I was so quiet, so deep down.*

I WANT *to be alive. I want to eat. I want to play. A woman I met in the infusion room who will be having a transplant next visited me and asked if I had short-term memory loss. If I do, I don't know it.* (I did.) *I do know I'm not sure what it will be like to be home again. Lying in bed, I look at people walking, oblivious to the fact that they are breathing so easily. As I hold on to the rail walking down the hall, I am proud of myself. But I get scared when I look at my body and see my flesh hanging there, like Mom's did when she was dying with lung cancer. Her lying in bed, unconscious and uncomfortable at the end of her life, is seared in my brain. But then I move my foot, I bend my leg, I wiggle my toes, exercising what I can. It helps me realize that I am 53, not 70. I have Mom's pluck and Dad's heart and David's love. Our love grows larger and larger. My time sitting and being with him is a gift. Precious. I know I am all right.*

October 24

I GO HOME TODAY! 5 WEEKS! *This has been "it," this small bright corner windowed room where I have observed wind/leaf/ temperature change from the inside. I've spent a lot of time gazing out the window at the sky. The room faces south and west. I see the sun setting and observe the changing colors, the movement of clouds, the hues of light, dark and bright, ever changing. Below is busyness, life moving, cars, people, trees. Looking out I feel my connection to the vastness of life, and the rhythm of nature. It is reassuring and calming.*

Lying here has been like a long retreat, only here I cannot leave and go outside. I focus on moving my body upright. Walking is an effort. I go slowly and not by choice, one foot and then the other. It's an achievement to walk up and down through the hall holding on to my IV pole and resting on David's arm. I feel good when I can move on my own, when I am awake. Today I was even able to watch a video, "Hello Dolly." I am alive . . .

Later . . . .

Nurses caring. David worrying. My stomach upset. Me quieter than I've ever been. I almost died. (It's a shock to realize how sick I was.) Now I know, yes, this can, does happen. I will die. I also know I want to recover. Please, let such danger be past for now. Let me heal. Let me get strong. May I have many good productive years with life, and with love. Give me time to be of service to others.

I feel Love as I sit still and warm with David . . . continuing to open our hearts to each other.

Teaching/Learning. Walking/Painting. Breathing in. Breathing out. Growing wiser.

May I use what I am learning selfishly and selflessly.
May we all be well.
May we all be free.
May each breath continue to be precious and appreciated.
May a sip of water hold its purity and the
miracle of quenching thirst.
May we be alive.
May we be free.
May we be here.
May we stay well.

Love helped me get through this experience. I thank every person who sent me wishes for healing. I don't know if the gratitude I feel can ever be fully expressed. The love I received was powerful motivation to stay alive and be well. May I be able to give back to others what they have so richly given to me.

SKY MEDITATION

The mind has been compared to the sky, vast and infinite. In this meditation you can begin by finding a seat either inside by a window or outside in a favorite spot that gives an expansive view of the sky. Be as comfortable as possible. If the weather is warm, you might even put a blanket on the ground and lie down, pillowing your head so you can comfortably sky-gaze.

BRINGING YOUR ATTENTION first to your breath and notice the rhythm of your breathing. Let your mind focus on the in-breath and the out-breath, perhaps even noticing the pauses between breaths. With eyes open, allow your eyes to sweep through the sky. Notice what captures your attention. Can you see the horizon? Where does the earth meet the sky? Are there any objects filling your frame of awareness? If so, be aware of its relationship to the sky. How much space does it occupy in your view of the sky? Move beyond the object, noting the play of light and color. What colors do you observe in the sky? Is it clear and blue or a dull grey? Is it the same color throughout? Are there clouds? If so, where are they located? What are their colors and shapes? Can you see them moving?

As you do this meditation, let yourself sit or lie back allowing the scene to come to you without striving to make something happen.

RESTING IN THE MOMENT, LET PEACE ABIDE.

If you like, as you end this meditation you can say and give to yourself: *"Peace above, Peace below, Peace inside. Peace all around. Peace. Peace. Peace."*

LOVING-KINDNESS MEDITATION

Doing this meditation has great benefits. It can help you experience joy and love, even rapture, helping us connect more intimately and authentically to ourselves and to others. Being loving and kind fosters compassion and understanding. It can sustain us in times of need.

To begin this meditation, make sure you have the time and are in a protected place. Pay particular care to your position; adjust it so that it is comfortable and will fully support your ability to let go and be held. The more you can trust this process and allow yourself to receive the well wishes of this meditation, the more potent it will be.

LET YOUR EYES CLOSE and allow yourself to relax. Notice the feelings in your body. Take a moment and be aware of any thoughts in the mind, or feelings. Simply let them be and watch them go like clouds floating along in a vast, blue sky. And if you'd like you can feel your breath moving in your body, a reminder that yes, you are here.

When you're ready, if you can, bring to mind an image of a person whom you've experienced as being loving and kind, a benefactor to you, someone who easily evokes feelings of warmth and love. To this person you can direct these phrases: *"May you be happy. May you be healthy. May you be safe and protected. May you live with ease."*

It is important that you connect to the meaning of the phrases. Feel free to substitute words of your own that resonate with you. Do this for a period of time until you feel a sense of the wishes that you are sending forth. When you feel ready you can move from giving these wishes to a benefactor to yourself. Wish yourself health and happiness, safety and ease of being. Take as much time as you like. If your mind wanders gently bring it back to the next phrase or repeat the one you had been saying. You can do this as often as you wish, adapting it so that it resonates with you, choosing words or phrases that have meaning for you that you can easily connect to as you say them to yourself. Take your time and say the phrases with love and intentionality repeating them slowly to yourself. Give them to yourself freely without straining or feeling guilty. The more full we feel and the happier we are the easier it is to radiate and reflect it out to others. Do this for as long as you want.

If you like, you can continue this meditation, sending the wishes for safety and protection, mental and physical happiness and ease of being to people in your life who are neutral to you, people that you may only see occasionally or even strangers. Notice what arises.

When you feel complete, almost like a pool being filled with love and kindness, compassion and joy, you can send these wishes to a difficult person. You can also send these wishes to parts of yourself that are hard for you to like and to accept. Do this with gentleness and care and only when you feel ready to do so.

You can continue repeating phrases of loving-kindness to yourself and others as often as you like, adding pets, plants, nature, all living and non-living beings, visible and invisible. You can do this wherever you are. The important thing is to feel the connection between yourself and the phrases, saying them with an open heart, tenderly and compassionately. Remember: be kind to yourself and do not judge. You are allowing yourself to ask for what you need and to receive these wishes, so you can be filled with peace. Then, you will be able to serve others as a beacon of peace and light.

WE'RE ALL IN THIS TOGETHER.
MAY WE ALL BE AT PEACE.

SECTION III

LISTENING AND WANTING

Listen. Listen.
To what you know.
Do not be lead by others though they be well
guided.

You know what is best.
Take your time.
Seek advice.
But listen to your self.

When it's time to go and do.
Do.
When it is time to rest.
Rest.

Listen.
And you will hear
Truth.

In truth I needed to rest, restore and replenish. Without really realizing it, I had fought a battle and now needed to recover. I was depleted physically, very anemic and needed frequent blood trans-

fusions. During my first week at home I couldn't even walk unaided.
I had to crawl up our stairs. There were no nurses to bring me a glass
of water and it was difficult for friends to visit. They had to be positive
that they were fully well. Even a slight cold could endanger my life.
I needed to be held but no one could touch me without wearing a
mask on their face or latex gloves. I was so tired and weak that I felt
like a little girl that needed her Mom. I missed my mother. In my
journal, I wrote:

SOMETIMES WE NEED TO BE SWADDLED IN LOVE.
SOMETIMES WE NEED TO BE SWADDLED IN LOVE.
SOMETIMES WE NEED TO BE SWADDLED IN LOVE.
SOMETIMES WE NEED TO BE SWADDLED IN LOVE.
SOMETIMES WE NEED TO BE SWADDLED IN LOVE.
SOMETIMES WE NEED TO BE SWADDLED IN LOVE
SOMETIMES WE NEED TO BE SWADDLED IN LOVE.

*Sometimes we need to hear Mommy, friend, beloved, respected
teacher say, "I love you, I think you're great."*
We can even say it to ourselves, You're Great! GREAT!!
TERRIFIC!!
And we need to believe this.
And take inside ourselves this favor
This love
This pleasure.
This sincerity of genuine care.

There is a time to spoil ourselves.
To be filled with honey and pomegranates and nectar.
To rest. To let go of striving.

You're great!
Yes, GREAT!
I'm writing this again and again.
It's important.
After a major exertion one needs to:

REST, RECOVER, RECUPERATE, RESTORE, REPLENISH
RETREAT, RECEIVE, RETURN HOME.

David was tired, too, and worried. He was back at work and came home exhausted. My brother arrived for a week to help out and spent the week taking me to the hospital for tests and transfusions and running errands. He indulged my cravings for forbidden foods like taco chips, although I discovered they were no longer tasty; my mouth was still so dry that it felt as if they were made of cardboard.

Suddenly, I couldn't tolerate mess. Everything had to be organized in my kitchen. One night, late, David and Bob made an emergency trip to the store for shelf organizers, which I then used late into the night, satisfying myself that my cans and kitchen goods were neatly categorized. I even had my brother rearrange the spices in my cabinet, labeling each one, and alphabetizing them. It helped me feel more in control. I wrote in my journal:

I am tired of having transfusions and worrying. I am tired of having to be so careful. I am tired. I wish this would all pass already. I am tired of being tired.

Writing this I wrap my blanket closer around me. I feel like a little girl helpless to boost my immune system and still dependent on others for so many basic necessities. I feel some self-pity. The dog, sensing this, curls up next to me.

As I grew stronger it seemed that my wanting mind also grew and with it came impatience and struggle.

I think a 'good' meditator would have equanimity and be non-attached. Instead I am sticky with impatience and lust for things to be different. How I wish to be happy and fulfilled instead of stopped up with clogged feelings, worry filling this moment with fear, craving what I can't have right now.

My wanting mind is busy thinking.

I am not content wearing a mask and having visitors have to wear a mask.

I know everything passes, but,

I lust for things to be different.
Not accepting
What is.

I will go.
Sit.
Quietly
Watching thought,
Feeling, breath,

  I might as well accept my wanting mind. NOW!

HERE'S MY LIST OF WANTS:

I want my body to be healthy and strong.

I want my husband to meet ALL my needs.

I want him to be emotionally available for me *whenever* I want.

I want appreciation and love.

I want every moment to count.

I want never to have self-doubt.

I want to be fulfilled, to be challenged, to be creative, to NEVER have down times.

I want to be physically coordinated and never fall.

I want discipline and spontaneity.

I want Mommy and Daddy, now dead, to put their arms around me.

I want Mommy to say, "I'm proud of you."

I want Daddy to make the mundane into a wonder
just like he used to do.

I want my brother and his family to be next door
so I can schmooze with them.

I want never to worry about my health.

I want to be content . . . to laugh and play more.

I want never to be tired in the middle of the day.

I want the stickiness of frustration and wanting to go away.

I want sadness to cease.

I WANT to be WELL.

WANTING IS OK. IT MEANS I AM ALIVE.
JUST HOLD IT LIGHTLY — BREATHE IN AND OUT —
LIGHT AND LOVE.

More Wants:
I want to be cured.
I want to be slim.
I want to feel sexy.
I want to like my body.
I want to feel fulfilled.
Why are my blood levels slow to come up?
I do not like being tired.
I do not like
WANTING.

EXERCISE: WANTING

This is an exercise that is best to do when you are actually feeling filled with frustration and aware of the gap between what you want and what you do or do not currently have. Instead of resisting this frustration, let yourself examine it more closely noticing how it is expressed in the body. Do you feel a constriction in your chest or your throat? Is there a tightness in your belly? Where are your shoulders now? Are they up by your ears or relaxed? What about your neck and back? Simply notice. Is there a sense of heaviness or tightness? Where? This exercise lends itself to non-verbal means of expression such as movement, writing and drawing.

TO GET READY, if you want you can select music that matches your mood and play it, stomping to the music or chanting "Oy Vey," or some other words that express how you are feeling. Then, when you are ready, choose your favorite art materials, get a large piece of paper or canvas and see if you can represent these angry, frustrated, negative feelings. If an image comes to you, draw it; if not let colors and form represent the feelings. Remember, this is for you. If you feel self-conscious, use your non-dominant hand for drawing. Have fun with this exercise; be creative. You can even use finger paints or clay. Do this as often as needed, noticing how your mood and feelings change in the process.

When you have completed your picture, take some breaths or get up for a moment or two and then sit down and look at it again. Then turn the paper over and write down whatever comes to mind, again without censoring any thoughts but letting them leave your mind and move onto the paper freely. If you like, you can time this exercise, writing freely for five minutes or however long you decide and then stopping.

EXERCISE: MY WANTS

Allow yourself to list your wants. Name and write them.

I want

I want

I want

I want

I want

Be aware of what thoughts, feelings and sensations arise as you do this. How is your breathing affected?

Review each "want" and imagine yourself blowing it into a bubble and watch it as it floats away. Observe the process noticing what arises as you watch it form and dissolve. Do this as many times as you like. Observe what happens as you let it go.

THANKSGIVING

Thanksgiving was approaching and I couldn't go to my aunt's house to celebrate with her and my cousins as I had often done in years past. My cousins are warm and funny and a link to childhood memories of large dinners and good times. I was disappointed, but still wanted to rejoice and give thanks for being alive. I decided I would make a big turkey dinner as a present for David and myself. I fantasized about cooking the turkey and making all the traditional dishes. I visualized myself tearing pieces of crispy skin off the turkey as I had when I was a kid. Mom would take the turkey out from the oven and I'd go to 'help' her and pick from the tray with the droppings. Delicious! I'd snack while Dad carved and he'd give me some especially juicy pieces. It was much better to eat it as it was being cut up rather than to be polite and wait.

On this Thanksgiving Day, I got up early to prepare the meal. It would be the first big meal I had made since before my hospitalization and I was excited. I decided to follow the turkey recipe from the *New York Times*. The author said that she had cooked nineteen turkeys and the nineteenth had been the best. She baked it at 500 degrees. The other instruction was, "No matter what, do not open the oven for 45 minutes."

I turned up the oven to 500 as I took out the turkey from the refrigerator. David worried that the turkey would grow bacteria while it was out of the refrigerator. He wanted to put the turkey in the oven right away. I worried that the oven wouldn't be hot enough unless we waited until it pre-heated. I needed to wait. He had a bad cold, was sniffling and uncomfortable and wore gloves and a tight mask over his face. I imagined the word WORRY painted on his forehead.

Both of us did our best to exercise restraint. In truth, I was too tired and in need of David to argue and he was too scared and too worried about losing me to make a fuss. I put the turkey in the oven, which seemed hot — very hot. After about twenty-five minutes, smoke began pouring out into the room and the smoke alarm went off. I was afraid to open the oven.

The smoke alarm is connected to our security system and automatically alerts the fire department. Urgently, frantically, we called the security people and tried to get them to cancel the alarm. It was too late. We opened all the windows and doors, put on our sweaters and waited until the oven cooled enough for us to open the oven door and put some water in the turkey pan to extinguish the small fire. Meanwhile, sirens blasting from the fire engine filled the air outside.

Two firemen quickly entered the house in their big rubber boots and hats. They saw the smoke, David in his mask, me with my bald head, and listened to our story. They were very understanding. They didn't laugh or berate me. I would have liked to have been able to offer them some turkey, but it still wasn't cooked. Was this a metaphor for my condition, I wondered: burned, but not done through and through?

Eventually, the turkey cooked and we could eat. It was not, however, the festive meal I had expected and once again I felt sad.

I feel like I'm in mourning for having to STOP, to STOP everything. I've had to STOP working and STOP my life, as I have known it. I'm being forced to be patient, to be my own client. I wish I could take a stress reduction class now. I'm feeling vulnerable and afraid.

As usual, when I was feeling upset and contracted, I realized I had to grow bigger, push down deeper, and come home to what was real and true. This need was a constant for me, going beyond any momentary thought, feeling or sensation. At the entrance to our house, David and I have a *mezuzah* nailed to the doorpost. It is on the right side, close to our hearts as we enter through the door. Mezuzah, in Hebrew, means doorpost. It is Jewish tradition to have one at the entryway of a home. It can also be placed in every doorway in the house. Tucked inside the mezuzah is a small piece of scroll on which is written, "Hear, Oh Israel, The Lord is God, God is One."

The tradition is to touch the mezuzah as one enters through the doorway. It is a way to connect to God, a reminder of unity and a presence larger than the self. It's also meant to protect the house and its occupants. It serves as a reminder to stop and be present. It says to me, "Wake up, perceive God and be held in love."

I needed to remember its message. Another reminder, in my tradition, is the Sabbath. On Friday night, candles are lit to indicate the separation of the workday from the day of rest. David and I do this each week. I light the candles and cup my hands and draw the light in, three times. Then we say the blessings and ask to be blessed. On that Thanksgiving, not a Sabbath, but a day of sadness and longing, I decided to give myself some blessings.

May the beauty within flower without.
May it be like milk from a mother to her child, plentiful and nourishing.
I am mother and child.

May I be blessed with peace and understanding.
May I have compassion for all my frailties.
May my determination be rooted in fertile soil,
giving strength to my heart.
May the thorns of my rose not cut into my own skin and
serve only to ward off harm.
May my sweetness be like honey to my soul.
May my awesomeness be free to soar and sing
without the need to hide.
May I dance under the sky and not worry that my belly is soft and
my neck has wrinkles.
May I have the energy to persevere and engage fully again and again.
May my creativity continue to burst forth like a spring of clear pure
water from which all may drink.
May I love myself and enter into my own garden of sunlight and
shade, impracticality and reason.
May I continue to love no matter what.
Then I am free.

Kadush Kadush Kadush
Holy, Holy, Holy

As time went on, I continued to jot down wishes for myself when I felt depleted or discouraged and needed a boost. The blessings served as inspiration and direction. Sometimes I repeated what I had written earlier. It didn't matter; my intention did. The desire to grow *and* be thankful rather than drown in frustration and sorrow motivated me and moved me towards positive goals.

Blessings: An Exercise

Below are some additional blessings that I gave myself. You may read them or skip ahead and write down your own blessings. You can do this at any time, all at once or as they come to you. You can give yourself a daily blessing and use it as a focus for the day. You can write this in your appointment book, journal, or a calendar. May it be a source of inspiration and hope.

My Blessings

May I be blessed with clarity of purpose.
May I be blessed with vision.
May I be blessed with joy and fulfillment.
May the flame of my passion for freedom burn steadily
like the burning bush,
Bright and beautiful without being consumed by self-pity.
May my vessel be strong,
my power pure and bright.
May my fears decrease or be useful as a guide rather than a block.
May I have the wisdom to see what is important and the courage
to follow what I know.
May my love flow and fill others and myself.
May my compassion to myself and others strengthen.
May I grace my humanness with loving-kindness smiles and
laughter,
May my shame cease and my wonder increase.
May I be free to be free and to embrace all that is there for me to
be whole.
May I not be ashamed to let my uncertainties show and my
openness and vulnerability be present.
May my beauty shine.
May I dance and sing and be free to grow.
May I be free.

Give Yourself Permission To Receive Your Own Blessings,
Letting Them Come Freely And Without Judgment.

GRATITUDE: A GUIDED MEDITATION

IN THIS MEDITATION, allow yourself to be filled with gratitude for the gifts you have received, the gift of life and the present of being able to be here now. With the in-breath, let yourself breathe in the joy of having a body and a mind. On the out-breath, let go and let yourself truly experience the miracle of release and surrender. You can let each cycle of breath be a reminder of the miracle of birth and death, endings and beginning.

Now allow yourself to open to the people in your life that have been good to you. Allow yourself to feel your love for them and thank them for their love and care. With each breath, as you feel or see these people in your mind's eye, let gratitude and appreciation grow.

Now when you are ready, let yourself review your life and the happenings that have helped you heal and grow, bringing happiness and wisdom. Allow yourself to give thanks. You may become aware of something that didn't happen and you can feel gratitude for being spared. Let yourself feel how fortunate you are, how rare it is to acknowledge your gifts. Give yourself permission to be filled with gratitude as you breathe with awareness and thanks for these gifts.

Now, is there anyone you would like to forgive, or ask for forgiveness? Let these persons, if any exist, come into your awareness. What about yourself? With each breath you may say, "May I be forgiven" or "I forgive you." And let that person (or traits) come clearly to mind. Tenderly notice the feelings that arise as you do this.

And when you have finished, knowing that this is a meditation than can be repeated as often as you like, you can expand your love and grace to include all people and all beings. May we all be here and held in love and peace.

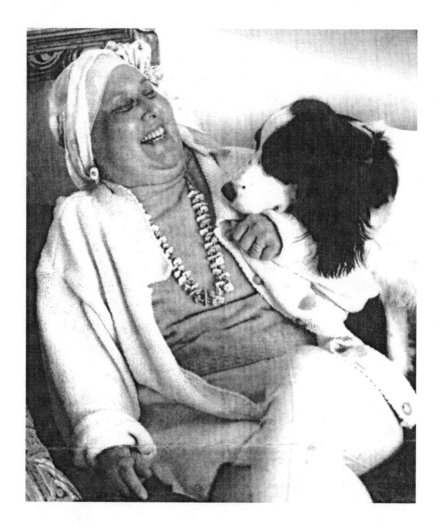

RE-ENTRY

The world has changed.
Yet it looks the same.
The tables, chairs, windows are in place.
Am I?

I breathe. I laugh. I cry.
It surprises me.
Others do the same.
They seem to take it as ordinary.

I am back.
But what now is normal?

I say to my classes.
WAKE UP!
To whom am I speaking?

I see courage. I see fear.

As I navigate the paths
of uncertainty, and difficulty,
can I
maintain a courageous heart?

The world has changed.
Or, have I?

Returning to work and resuming a more active lifestyle was BIG, so big in fact that I could only address it indirectly. Without realizing it, my close encounter with death and the strength it took to maintain my equanimity had changed me. My mind was working to make meaning of the experience and processing it took time. My cousin had written a personal credo for a ceremony in the Unitarian church, which inspired me to write down mine. I did it, simply letting my thoughts flow. In retrospect, I realize that I was summing up my experience and preparing myself to re-enter society.

MY CREDO

Some people after a great battle go on to the next one, that being their duty and chosen vocation. Others choose to go home to rest and recuperate until they must fight again. I choose to fight only battles of mind that hinder clarity and wisdom. It is tempting to forget or deny my nearness to death. I do not want to relive the difficulties of my hospitalization and recuperation. I resolve to dwell in the present and not be captured by fear. I shall use my experience to remember the preciousness of life and the gifts I have received. I shall challenge myself to live wisely and make meaning of my experience, letting it transform me. I shall work to bring peace to others, so they too, may, be free. I am filled with gratitude to all who have helped me be alive and well. May I never forget the grace that has been bestowed upon me.

There is a sense of urgency to accomplish my goals but I shall not act in haste or imprudence. I shall listen and do what my soul knows is important, without needing to know whether I shall see the harvest of my labors.

It is not important what will be tomorrow. It is important to live today in harmony with myself and others and to use the love I receive to give it out again. I must act from wisdom and not let impatience lead me to deception and infirmity.

I shall work to maintain a balance, opening to what is true and acting accordingly. I shall not be ashamed of praise, but value my efforts, appreciate my bravery and celebrate my joy. May I be able to: Enjoy; Replenish; Dance and Sing; Make love; Care fully for the body and the spirit and help others do the same.

Clearly, my brush with death had changed me, but I was still digesting my experience. How it would affect me was unknown but my intentions were clear. I knew that I wanted every moment to count. I was aware of my impatience to move on and had to be patient. This wasn't easy. I couldn't wait to get out of the house and be in public places again; I even looked forward to going to the supermarket and being able to choose my own supplies of dishwasher soap, fruits, vegetables and frozen goods. Going out to a restaurant and choosing from a menu of delights felt like a dream, my nirvana. I didn't know how my work-life would be affected. I wanted to sing, dance, make love and be happy.

Nothing is permanent; to my relief that included my quarantine. David and I decided to go to Northern Italy to celebrate my re-entry into the world. It was early spring and the weather in New England was still cold, but in Tuscany and Umbria and along the coast in Cinque Terre it was warm and filled with bright colors, sunshine and the ambient Italian life. It was almost as if I had entered into the poster that had for so long sat propped up against the wall, warming up my hospital room. We leisurely explored Northern Italy. I tired easily so we went at a slow pace, stopping for long lunches accompanied by a bottle of wine. Each day when I needed to rest, we paused in a park with a beautiful vista or sipped lattes in a cafe. We lunched in the mountains and by the sea. It was *La Dolce Vita*. All was *bella*.

I was in love. I was in love with Italy, David, and the freedom of being able to explore and be out in the world again. All of my senses were engaged. Every mouthful of food — and there were many — tasted extraordinarily delicious. The fruit and vegetables were fresh and juicy and beautiful to look at. My diet had been so limited for so long. "The hell with my weight," I thought. We had two three to five course meals every day and I loved each one.

I savored every moment, every step, every site. We rented a small Fiat and David, pretending to be a race car driver, drove like a fiend, (or an Italian). I was proud of his ability to weave in and out of traffic and take the narrow curvy roads as he lifted his foot from the clutch and the brake.

During this trip he was very protective of me. Was I warm enough? Did I need to stop and rest? Normally his long legs would take him two or three strides ahead of me and I'd have to run or yell out, "Slow down." Here he held my hand and we walked together. I appreciated having him with me, relaxed and relatively unworried. The trip was a wonderful break for both of us, taking us away from doctors, hospitals and the reminders of cancer. I came home refreshed and ready, at last, to return to work.

The Stress Reduction Clinic had moved in the time that I had been away, now sharing space with the research wing of Behavioral Medicine on the top floor of a building close to the medical center. Each office had a window and for the first time I now had my own space. I remember walking into the building for the first time and entering the corridor where a staff meditation had just begun. Every person on the staff was sitting quietly, either on a cushion or a chair, in the hallway between our offices. There was a seat set aside for me, which I took as I closed my eyes and entered into the silence of the meditation. As I felt my breathing, I became aware of warmth in the area of my heart. A deep sense of gratitude and awe filled my chest. My eyes teared up. Being able to walk up the stairs and sit with my dear friends and colleagues in the clinic felt very special, something I could never take for granted.

My first teachers' meeting was also wondrous. As I joined the circle my colleagues and I formed, I felt at home, but very new to the experience. It was almost as if I were a baby emerging from its swaddling cloth, arms and legs now released to explore the world without being bound. What a miracle to be here. I saw with fresh eyes and appreciated anew the wonder of life.

It was arranged that Fernando DeTorres would share the teaching with me for my first cycle of classes. Fernando had put a string around his wrist as soon as he heard I needed a transplant; on our first day of class together, he ceremoniously took it off.

On Memorial Day, about six weeks after I started working again, I wrote the poem that appears on the next page. It reflected the euphoria I was experiencing.

It is morning in the springtime.
May 24.
Memorial Day Weekend.

Spring is late this year.
I am here.

I am not having chemo.
My hair is growing.
The dogwood is blooming and the ash trees are budding at last.

I look out my window and it is green.
My husband sleeps.
Yes.

I am alive. What wonder.
How full it is

To use my mind
To reclaim my body
To celebrate the moment

Breathing in and out.

I do not know when my breath will cease.
I do know I love.
I love the day,
The people in my life.
I love
Being Here Now.

I plunged into activities. I was no longer falling when I walked. I even had hair. It was very short and showed off my eyes. I loved feeling it on my head and not needing scarves or hats to protect me from the sun. I still tired easily, but I was able to go to the gym and work out to regain greater strength and muscle tone. I got myself a personal trainer, Cheryl Mita, who consistently buoyed my spirit and helped me be positive about my progress. It was very important to me to restore my muscles and increase my aerobic capacity. I went to the gym several times a week and as I was able to exercise for longer periods of time and my repetitions increased on the machines my sense of accomplishment grew.

Yet, how easy it is to forget to be present. Just today I looked in the mirror at myself and called myself "ugly" because my face is still puffed up from the prednisone I had to take. I didn't say to myself, "What a miracle, I'm breathing without an oxygen mask . . . I am able to stand . . . my hair is growing back! . . . I am alive!" Instead I focused on the puffiness of my face and suffered needlessly.

Teaching helped normalize some of my frustration with the slowness of my recovery. As I coached others to be present and make peace with their difficulties, I was encouraged to hang in with my own. Class came to an end in June and I prepared to teach the summer session class, my first one teaching alone since I had begun treatment for cancer. It was my first summer without chemotherapy in two years.

A film crew from "Chronicle," a news show on the local ABC station, was coming to the clinic to tape some classes and document the work we were doing in stress reduction. My class was selected as the one they would feature and follow for eight weeks. This made me extra nervous, both for myself (How would I look?) and for the class. I was concerned about confidentiality and the intrusion of a film crew on our class process. I wondered if patients would be free to report honestly on their progress in meditation and truly express their deepest concerns.

The film crew was sensitive and only featured those people who wished to appear on TV. I still worried that the class's integrity might be compromised or my teaching might not be up to par (and that everyone would see it). Fortunately, I focused so closely on the patients that I forgot to be self-conscious and we all got used to having microphones and booms in the room. I was reminded, once again, that as long as I was *really present,* there was no problem. When the producers discovered that I had recently had a peripheral stem cell transplant for lymphoma, I became part of the story.

At one point during the program, the commentator asked, "What qualifies someone to teach others how to overcome fear and pain?"

And the commentator answered, "In the case of Elana, experience."

The cameras moved to the bone marrow unit in the hospital, illustrating and describing the procedure by showing footage of a patient currently on the unit. The interviewer visited me at home and borrowed some photos of me taken when I had just come home from the hospital, showing me with clear eyes, a puffy face, and looking pale and ill.

They also interviewed my hemo-oncologist, Dr. Pam Becker, who surprised me by saying, "The staff watched in awe as Elana brought herself through an incredible amount of physical stress which was very demanding."

The program recorded footage of several class members who had particularly moving stories: a single mother as she helped her child who had muscular dystrophy climb up a stair; an older man who had had a heart attack listening to the body scan on earphones as he sat by his boat; and another single mother talking about how difficult it was raising her children alone as she struggled financially after recovering from drug addiction.

Patients were shown in class, meditating, doing a body scan and yoga. In a discussion regarding the difficulty of practice, they captured me as I said, "Of course you're going to have a struggle. Just know it, it's normal. Struggle isn't a problem; getting stuck in it is."

When I was asked what I had learned from my own experiences that was useful to my teaching, I paused and spontaneously said, "Waking up and feeling terror. It was hardest for me to accept I was afraid. I am now more understanding toward fear."

And I suggested to the audience, "Trust yourself; be more in the present moment. Stay with direct experience rather than anticipating problems even with a disease that is difficult to accept and is painful. That way you can have a full life. And," I repeated confidently, "You *can* have a full life."

Class ended. The film crew left and I breathed many sighs of relief as I prepared to enjoy my fuller life, returning again to the beach for our vacation. Once again, Bekka would spend a week with us. This time, there was no hospital, no chemotherapy and no restrictions. Only joy. I could swim in ponds again. I could eat out. There were no catheters. I still got tired, but I could nap.

Every morning, David and I rose early and took our dog, Chaya, to the beach for her daily run. I noticed that each day I could go a little bit longer. Life seemed to be resuming a more normal pace.

EXERCISE: MY CREDO

I wrote my credo in stages. At first, I used the third person and wrote in flowery language. It was too painful to say "I" and own my feelings. As time passed, I was able to go back, review what I had written and adjust it to reflect more accurately how I wanted to live.

LET YOUR ATTENTION settle on your breath, letting everything go but this moment and the sensations of breathing. Allow yourself to open to your experience now, witnessing it without judgment and letting it move through you with the breath. Give yourself as much time as you need for the mind to quiet.

When you feel settled you can ask yourself, *"What is my credo? What are the guidelines for my life?"*

Ask yourself if they are really your guidelines or ones imposed upon you. Let your credo come to you, giving it time and space to know what rings true. You can inquire deep inside yourself asking, *"What do I believe? How does it color my actions?"*

Jot down some thoughts and look at them again. This exercise is useful to do more than once, at different times and dates. Use it for reflection and learning, and when you're ready, write it out fully. It can serve as a mission statement, a goal to work towards and a source of inspiration and courage. Base it on strengths and aspirations, converting weaknesses into possibilities for growth.

SEASONS CHANGE

Every moment is a precious moment.
The leaves fall
orange, red, brown.
Some still fresh and shiny.
Each color varies.
Each shape unique.
among the sameness of type.

My eyes close.
I see leaves, shapes
and colors,
maple and oak.

This year I melt paraffin.
I want to preserve the beauty
of the leaf.

I know it has died
I know it will not stay forever.
Yet, it is here now
and beautiful.

I enjoy
looking.
Breathing in the air.
Crisp. Fresh.

The stars shine bright.

I sink down into sleep,
thankful,
trusting,
I shall wake
to live another day.
to give,
to receive.

as I tend
with tenderness
the stream of life
and watch
the seasons change.

FALL

I wanted to hold on to joy, this freshness of being and wonder that opened my eyes anew, but I couldn't. A cornerstone of Buddhism is impermanence. Many times I told myself, "Cling to nothing and you shall be happy."

However, I am accomplished in holding on and not letting go. I was invested in staying well and not having a recurrence. My mind knew that I couldn't hold on to my health or my new aliveness of spirit any more than the leaf could stay attached to the tree. Yet I still felt sad, anticipating the oncoming darkness of winter and the possibility of a recurrence of cancer.

I read *Freddy the Leaf*, a children's book about dying, written by Leo Buscalia. In it, we get to know Freddy, a large, healthy leaf, as he takes his place on a tree with other leaves. Freddy loves being part of the tree. It provides shade for the children and the elderly and is very lovely. When the winter wind arrives and carries his friends away he doesn't want to go. A wise leaf tells him this is a natural process, but still Freddy holds on. One day a strong wind comes and he falls gently to the ground and rests on the snow. It is peaceful. We learn the snow will melt and will help feed the tree for another season.

I used to read this story in the fall because it is the time when my mother was very ill with lung cancer. I vividly remember her fear of dying and wish to hold on. On Rosh Hashanah, the Jewish New Year, she was very weak and only with difficulty could she rise from her bed. Traditionally, each year her "group," friends she had known all her married life who had grown up with my father from his Hebrew School days, had a party to celebrate the New Year. These friends were very important to her, so much so that she asked two of the boys, men in their early forties, to come to the house and carry her to the party.

I shall never forget the sight of my mother being lifted from the bed onto a small chair. It wasn't steady and she had very little strength, but she gripped its sides tightly and held on as it tottered, high in the air. When she got to the party she was sweaty and exhausted. She sat down, smiled and quickly tore off her wig. She was pale and couldn't eat, but she glowed. She had made it. Three weeks later she died.

Like my mother, I was determined to do all that I could to live fully until I died, and to do what was under my control to stay well. I read David Spiegel's book, *Living Beyond Limits,* which describes how he discovered, to his surprise, that women who were in support groups tended to have longer periods of remission then those who were not. This data inspired me to organize a support group of other women who had had transplants. One of the coordinators at the transplant unit gave me some names of people whom she thought might be interested. It turned out that each woman was associated with the medical center in some way and each was very active and dynamic. Cancer wasn't stopping us, but it had changed our lives and altered us. As one of the women said, "There aren't too many people you can talk to about worries and have it be normalized and not blown out of proportion."

The first meeting was at my house. None of us had known each other prior to transplant. I had met Agnetha in the waiting room before chemotherapy sessions. She had recommended the transplant unit at the University of Massachusetts Medical School to me and seen me on the unit prior to her own transplant. She recalls I gave her a thumbs up sign as I walked down the hallway in the unit. Linda is a cardiologist at the hospital and had been called in on a consult with me, neither of us suspecting that soon she would be there herself for a recurrence of lymphoma. Janet, Ann and Peggy had breast cancer, the rest of us lymphoma. We were all around the same age, but quite different, with different backgrounds and occupations. None of us wanted cancer to be the focus of our lives and we were all living with uncertainty more consciously than a person who hadn't been touched by a life-threatening illness. Linda coined the name for our group, "Stem Cell Sisters."

Ann Nemitz, a family physician, was the first of our group to have a recurrence. Aware of the limits of her time, she used her condition and position in the medical school to create a curriculum for medical students on end of life care that was both sensitive and practical. As she taught medical students how to be with the dying, she met each of her own medical crises with courage and strength. Her ability to stay clear and meet each new moment as it came with equanimity while remaining considerate of others and their needs was a source of inspiration to us all, family, friends, and the larger medical community. She even thought to make videos for her daughter, Megan, still in college, to be viewed when she got married and at the birth of her baby.

While Ann was still well enough to think clearly, she gathered her close friends and family around her and planned for her end of life care. She wished to die as consciously as possible. She and I sat and meditated together with a picture of the medicine Buddha in front of us. Ann prepared us for her death by her frankness and fearlessness. She enriched my life. I miss her.

We stem sisters don't like to think of ourselves as a high risk group. In truth, cancer does not take center stage when we meet, but we are aware that every moment counts.

WINTER

First snow
David shoveling it away.
Outside trees are bare.
Inside it is warm.

A blessing to be alive and to watch
whiteness blanket the trees.
Snow fills the shovel.
A path is made.

Trees are in dormancy now
Yet they stand erect.
Cancer cells sleep too . . . I hope.
I prepare to exercise.
To work my body.
To be strong.
I am in love
With
The comings and goings.
The messiness/beauty of life
as we are here in it

Now.

The leaves I had so carefully tried to preserve in September were drying and fading. I was engaging in more activities, but I was concerned about my energy level. I worried that I might not have enough to sustain me through the next session of class. I was assigned interns. We would meet immediately after the class ended to discuss what happened. This was a two-and-a half-hour session, which followed a two-and-a half-hour class. This brought my teaching time up to five hours. Five hours of pure concentration and being "on." I wasn't sure I could manage this. The interferon I was taking to boost my immune system was causing flu-like symptoms and increased my fatigue. It also caused joint pain. I felt like a 90-year-old woman who needed help getting out of her chair. Now it was an effort to be awake and lively if it was late in the day.

On the days that I taught my stress reduction class, I would come home and immediately go to bed. If I took an aerobics class, I'd have to have a nap or be very tired the rest of the day. I felt my fatigue most adversely affected my home life. David came home around 7:00 p.m. We'd eat and, from my perspective, have a desultory conversation. By the time David wound down from work, I'd either be asleep or ready for bed. He never complained and seemed very appreciative of having me alive and with him. I, however, was sensitive to the fact that my libido had not really recovered and I wished that my zest and passion would return. The trees were in dormancy. Was my body slowed down so it could regenerate, too?

In January, a routine CAT scan showed small spots on my lungs.

There are dots on my chest of unknown origin or etiology. A lung biopsy is required.

"*Oh, no.*"

I do not want this. This requires surgery, being in the hospital again, perhaps a six-week recovery. That is, if everything is all right. My strength is just beginning to return. I am back at work teaching again — just beginning to find a new rhythm.

I didn't believe that I had lung cancer or metastasis, but it had to be ruled out. TB tests were negative. There was no explanation for what could be causing these spots. Our friend the hematologist said, "It's probably just debris, things like this happen. Who knows?"

Hans Selye defined stress as "wear and tear." I was now experiencing wear and tear as I went for X-rays, CAT scans, Gallium scans, breath tests, etc. As I sat in meditation I realized that I was upset. I didn't fear death. I didn't want to have to go through all the tests. I hated the thought of having my chest opened up. I was just beginning to feel confident and comfortable at work, my strength slowly increasing in spite of the fatigue.

My friend, Agnetha, who had had a transplant shortly after mine and stayed in the same corner room, discovered what appeared to be the same spots in her lungs. She thought it might have been a fungus which we had inhaled while in the hospital. It was very tempting to ignore the spots but we were afraid not to know if they were lethal so we elected to have the exploratory surgery.

The surgeon was a lovely man. He had a Scottish accent and a soft voice. When he saw me meditating as I waited for him in the examining room, he expressed an interest in it. He told me he admired my calm. Calm? I thought. I'm still and I'm quiet, but calm? He was as reassuring as he could be, telling me he'd try to use a scope and only make four small incisions. If this didn't work, he'd have to open my chest to take a sample of whatever was there.

I felt very fatalistic as I went into the hospital. I remember stowing my street clothes in a locker and putting on the hospital johnny. Tying the skimpy cloth of the robe together brought back bad memories. I worried about the anesthesia. I feared having a large incision and a slow recovery. I didn't let my mind think about finding more cancer. Instead, I focused on the surgery and tried not to anticipate problems.

When I woke up in the recovery room. The surgeon stood by the bed, smiling. "No cancer," he said. And he had been able to do the work he needed with a scope. Relief. Joy. Exuberance. A few weeks later, Agnetha, too, got a clean bill of health.

In the Hospital 1/9/98
Outside,
gray rain
spattered window.

Inside,
white sheeted bed.
I am tired
but at rest.

Good news makes me uncomfortable
but
I like it–
A LOT.

No cancer.
No treatment for cancer.

I can heal and live more days
more nights.

Listen to more stories.
Turn the key to the ignition
On.

Wash my face.
Brush my hair.
Make plans for the future.

My incision hurts but
I know
It is healing.

I have survived.
I say, "Thank God."

A week later, I went off to Florida to be with my husband's aging parents, Gertrude, 85, and Morris, 91. Morris was having difficulty walking. He had survived two bouts of lymphoma, the first over 20 years ago, and now had a small nodule that seemed cancerous in his lungs. He probably also had prostrate cancer and had to urinate frequently, waking him throughout the night. He refused any more medical treatment.

Morris was the patriarch of the family. He had supported his younger brother and two sisters after their father and mother had died young. He took over the family business, a grocery store, and always worked long and hard, priding himself on his strength and capacity for work. David remembers him carrying crates and hoisting large carcasses of meat as he did his own butchering. Now he was limited in his activities. He felt weak and didn't like it. He had no feeling in his feet and it was painful for him to walk. He spent much of the day sitting in his chair in the living room, working the remote and watching TV. The sound was turned up loud, as he was hard of hearing.

Religion was important to Morris, especially since he had retired and had the time to go to synagogue and say the daily prayers. Now that he was homebound he would take out his prayer book and *tefillin*. (Thin leather straps that you wrap around you, one to hold a small box on the forehead with the *Shema* written inside, "Hear O Israel, The Lord our God, The Lord is One," and the other to be wrapped around your left arm, closest to your heart.) Morris put on the teffilin and *davened* (prayed) each day, morning and evening. He said he did this to bring God into his heart and give thanks for still being alive.

I valued this practice, but I also felt shut out from it. Morris was a strong, quiet man but he felt separate from the rest of us. His presence was huge but I never quite knew how to get close to him. I was used to parents who yelled and cried and laughed. I was not used to silence or the tension of repressed feelings.

It seemed to me that David's mother centered all her activities around Morris's needs. She'd consult him for any decision and wait on him. She wasn't feeling well herself and was having dizzy spells and stomach pain but she never complained. (I love to *kvetch* [complain]). This too, made me uncomfortable.

The condo was very small and it was very hot and humid. We couldn't turn the air conditioner up to make it cooler because Morris didn't like that. Then the air conditioner broke and David had to take his mother, Gert, to the hospital for tests. This left me alone with Morris and his aide in this hot, humid, cramped space. I felt I had to remain to be present for the repairman. I was sweaty and uncomfortable. The aide decided to complain to me. My equanimity, already strained by my own surgery, vanished, as did my sense of compassion. I was drowning in self-pity, irritability and frustration.

When David and Gert got home we planned to go to a nice, cool restaurant for a family dinner, perhaps the last time we might be able to do this together. Gert asked Morris to put in his hearing aid. He would not. She asked him a few times and he repeatedly said, "No."

This was too much for me.

"We want to be able to talk to you," I yelled. "I won't go if you won't put it in."

No one ever fought Morris this directly. The room was silent. Then Morris blew up at me.

"I'm a dying man."

And then I lost it. Heatedly, I retorted, "I'm younger than you are and I could die, too."

Pause.

"We want to be with you at dinner and talk with you," I said.

I retreated to the back room, shaken. Morris began to cry. David and his mother did nothing and said nothing. Clearly, I had gone beyond acceptable behavior. I cooled down and apologized for not being respectful. Morris put in his hearing aid and we went out to eat. We returned home and I wrote this poem.

Fear arises.
I am in Florida
With my 91 year old father-in-law.
He is now disabled.
Hard to walk. Hard to hear.

I suggest a hearing aid.
He replies,
"What for?"

We both pray.

Being in the present moment.
                    Facing wholly what is here.
Holy. Whole.

I am aware of
The courage to hear, to see, to think to feel, to live
and to experience with ALL *my senses*
as my Daddy told me.

It takes wisdom to know when to avert eyes.
When not to push.
Is it kindness or compassion
to be silent?

Suggesting nothing
Respecting the wish to STOP.
Listening.

Right now,
My chest hurts.
I have scarring in my lungs.

How can I keep an open heart and be holy whole?

Morris, at ninety-one, couldn't change. Both of us were feeling sorry for ourselves. Both of us were angry and hurt. How sad that we couldn't connect and comfort each other.

SPRING

Be Kind to Your Pain

Be kind to your pain
Touch it lightly
Kiss the hurt with your heart
Soothe it with faith.

You are all right.
Simply trust.
Surrender.

Then there is no problem.

The body decays.
When the mind is Awake
There is no problem.

We are whole.

Have faith.
You are held.

Everything passes.

Spring is a time of year when new life bursts into bud and normally brightens my mood. David and I were married in the springtime. We had forsythia wound around the poles that held up our *chupah*, canopy, under which we married. Now the forsythia was blooming again, but sadness still lingered. Fatigue continued to be a problem, forcing me to acknowledge my vulnerability. I also felt time ticking away. I knew self-mastery had to be now, not tomorrow, but I felt clogged with grief. Moving on required working with my grief and disappointment. It was very humbling to acknowledge my own inadequacies, anger, frustration and self-pity. Teaching stress reduction continued to inspire me, but it also seemed to point out discrepancies

between my ideal self — wise, calm, and unperturbed by fatigue —
and the self that struggled with exhaustion. Just when I thought I
reached a state of equanimity and had things figured out, something
would change, a physical symptom or an emotional snag. I knew it
was time for me to go on retreat again.

I chose a loving-kindness, Metta retreat. I thought it would be
useful to spend ten days to cultivate a quiet mind and an open heart
filled with love and compassion.

February 1998: On Retreat
*Who knows what will be? I am happy to be here now, breathing,
walking, smiling.*

*I cannot forget when this was not possible. It is very precious to love
and be loved and to appreciate each moment. I consciously sip vegetable
broth and taste its flavor. I am awake and aware and can concentrate,
even write in my journal.*

*Do I worry? I do. But as I rest my head on my 26-year-old sleeping
bag that is soft and fluffy and filled with down, I am at peace and
happy. I feel safe and protected and at ease. Equanimity now is no
problem. Bubbling inside like a geyser almost ready to pop is Joy.*

*The wonder of it all, (being alive and able to care for myself) even
brushing my teeth.*

The bell rings.

*So short a day is. My sense of time is altered. The evening comes
and the sky darkens. Just moments ago light shone on this spot which
now is dark. I listened to a talk by Sylvia* [Sylvia Boorstein, a meditation
teacher] *on zeal. She described how in the face of a tsunami in Hawaii
she and others sat on the roof of the meditation hall watching and
waiting for it, holding hands and being stalwart and* VERY AWAKE
*as they faced the possibility of imminent disaster. The giant wave never
came but as they left, relieved, thinking they were safe, the nearby
volcano erupted. "There's always something," said Sylvia.*

Wednesday 11:20 a.m.
*Instruction: Send Metta to an enemy, someone who is difficult for
you or whom you don't like. I picture my difficult person. I do not like
her. As I connect to her in my mind, I feel my own obstinacy and*

resistance. I realize I am a package of dynamite and she has as much difficulty with me as I do with her.

I feel my energy accelerate like a newly charged battery ready for use. I walk off some of the energy, return to the room and write:

I give thanks
to these moments
of sun
shining.

Warmth, light, vitality
the ability to walk and trot
to work up a sweat.
To have energy.
I am full
as my body balances
and legs move.

The refreshment of a shower.
The exuberant vibrancy of insight.

Joy.
In recognition
of power, health
and being
a little dynamo.

As I feel the energy of my own willfulness I realize what a handful I must have been to Mom. Realizing this allows much of the old anger I had towards her to melt. She has been more difficult for me to forgive than the person I chose to send Metta and forgiveness toward. Focusing on love brings up old pain.

Mom, now I understand. You were afraid, hurt, too scared yourself, too fearful of what could go wrong to appreciate my natural joy. Too worried, expecting another catastrophe. Being the second youngest of eight kids and poor, and your Mom angry and overworked, you didn't know you were loved.

Yet, Mom, Goldie, kept alive a spark, glimmers of spirit shimmering with her smile, her laugh, her tenderness and kindness, her vulnerability.

She was soft and warm, wonderful to hug. She made me feel good as well as bad. I felt safe and protected, loved, not only criticized. And she married my father, "Smilin Jack." He certainly wasn't practical but he had charm and exuberance. "I'm Jack's wife," she would say proudly.

I am Goldie's daughter. I have her warmth, her ease with people, her insight and intuition. Metta to myself is to say good-by to her sadness and the heavy weights of her disappointments. They are not mine. I can replace fear with caution and not be ruled by it. I can conquer cancer and take joy in being alive.

Hearing the melting snow drip outside my window.
My hair wet and freshly shampooed.
My cheeks still pink from my walk.
My clothes fresh.
My belly moving with my breath.

Sitting and writing and feeling secure
Here
in my room at IMS.
I am content.

With understanding comes release and rest.

Evening Talk
    Sharon Saltzberg talked about compassion and sympathetic joy, being happy for another.

    Sharon reminds me of my brother Bob so I call him. I am being indulgent to myself on this retreat. He has been on retreat and has also had some insights about our mother. He sounds sad. "You can be happy," I tell him. It feels like a major discovery.

    "Bubble on," says he.

    I feel a little sad as I hang up the phone. It is dangerous talking to another while on retreat. I am vulnerable and sensitive. I feel the distance of our two experiences in this moment. I love him and his family and they are far away.

    I go in the kitchen to get my Chinese herbal tea. Sylvia Boorstein is there. I give her a big smile and she smiles back. Happiness again. Joy! She reminds me of the best of my mother. It's OK to be happy. HAPPY!

I appreciate my husband for appreciating my spirit. He's my booster.
Bubbles and dynamite.
Sadness and Joy.
"It's OK to be happy."
Having the luxury of retreat and the time and safety to watch it all
come and go, healing the self, repairing the hurts, allowing the glow of
completeness to be experienced. Riding it all, is that equanimity?

To my niece Bekka, 2/11/98
I am sitting here on my bed on retreat, eating a cookie, and making
crumbs all over. It is good. I am cultivating joyous thoughts. I am having
a revelation of something you already know. It's wonderful to be happy.
I am happy. I bubble away in joyous thoughts and feelings. I feel a lot of
love all around me, from you, teachers, and the other men and women
sitting here quietly and repeating to themselves, "May I be happy. May
I be free. May I be safe and protected. May I have ease of being."

It makes me remember watching Peter Pan *on Broadway with my*
mother and father. "Think happy thoughts," said Peter to the lost boys,
instructing them in flying. And later . . . as Tinker Bell's light dims, he
beseeches the audience to clap if they can believe in fairies. "Clap!" he
says, "Clap!" and as we do, her light shines anew. Believe!

The air is fresh with moistness
I celebrate my life.
You are here.

As the moon illuminates the night
My heart fills
with light
and happiness.

Tea Time, Monday
Sitting outside, contentedly licking my peanut butter sticky fingers,
I realize what a miracle it is to be here, content and present. It takes me
by surprise to realize I can feel this way whether I wait in line to wash
my dishes or I sit in the meditation hall, noticing that my posture isn't
comfortable and wanting to move.

In an interview the teacher asked, "Why are you here?"

I am here for hope. Here for patience. Here to help each moment be experienced with greater equanimity. I am here to be with friends, my community, and feel the support, and the shared desire to be free from old conditioning and to be happy. I am here to heal, to hear the birds, the chipmunks, to observe the green shelled hardness of the pine cones. Here to feel my toes and the soles of my feet touch the bottom of my shoe or the slippery coolness of the polished wood floor . . . Here to be more alive . . . to feel peace . . . to be free from wanting to be elsewhere or for the moment to be different than it is.

I returned from retreat inspired and looking forward to being away again on another retreat in just two weeks, with Kamala Masters and Steve Armstrong in Hawaii. Kamala had sat with me in the hospital when I was sick. She had been able to be with me when I was so far away and close to death. Her presence now reminded me of the peace she had brought with her into the high tech sterile atmosphere of my hospital room and inspired me.

It was very special to sit a retreat in Hawaii. The retreat was held in a converted bed and breakfast inn halfway up the volcano in Maui and overlooking the waters of the bay. Greenery surrounded us. The temperature was inviting and I had a room in the main house that I shared with two others. I got the big bed. The food was wonderful and we could eat sitting on the veranda which overlooked the bay. The environment was so beautiful and lush I felt overwhelmed and awed to be there.

One morning, in an interview with Steve, I told him how happy I was feeling and how the beauty of the place seemed to fill me. "Well, you know who lives here?" he asked.

Immediately the Garden of Eden came to mind.

"Snakes?" I blurted out.

Steve laughed and said, "No, gods."

That never would have occurred to me. It was a wonderful reminder not to anticipate trouble.

Meditation On Compassion

It's often easy to be loving and kind to others but often more difficult to be compassionate to ourselves. This meditation is designed to bring compassion to our own pain and suffering. To begin this meditation get into the position that gives you the greatest sense of comfort and ease yet allows you to remain awake and alert. Choose a time to do this when you can be free to be alone and uninterrupted, without any "have to's" lingering in your mind. It is wise to do this in a warm and comfortable place that you now associate with relaxation and renewal, a sanctuary that you have created that is pleasing and supports your ability to experience peace.

WHEN YOU ARE READY, you can bring your awareness to your breathing or say to yourself the phrases of Metta, *"May I be safe and protected, May I be happy, May I be healthy, May I live with ease."* If it is easiest for you to connect to the phrase by first sending these wishes to a person who has been a benefactor to you, do so. When you feel that your attention has stabilized and your mind has quieted, then send these wishes to yourself.

As you are ready, you can add, *"May I bring compassion to my pain."* You may also say this phrase alone.

It is important that you can access the feeling that compassion brings, perhaps by recalling a time you felt compassion toward another person. Let the warmth, care and sympathy that arises with compassion be felt and send it into the areas inside of you that need this tender touch of kindness. You can focus it around the heart center and, if you like, imagine compassion being pumped down through the body and into the mind. Really, let compassion fill your awareness as you allow the wounds of heart and mind to be swathed in love and care.

If it is helpful, you can add music to this meditation, the in-breath bringing in compassion and care and on the out-breath releasing resistance and struggle.

May you be free from suffering.

May you be compassionate and kind.

May you open to beauty and love.

May you be compassionate to yourself and your struggles.

May you be free.

Give yourself permission to be receptive to the loving-kindness of compassion. Feel free to improvise as you open and soothe the hurts that block happiness and freedom. Remember, this is for you; there is no need to judge what arises, whatever appears, honor it with compassion and love. You deserve it. If you like, you can include loved ones, sending compassion to them, and then let yourself receive it back, noting the thoughts, feelings and bodily sensations that develop as you do this meditation.

When it is time to end, gently wiggle fingers, and toes and move your body; opening your eyes to meet the next moment with greater kindness and hope.

CHALLENGE: "I WON'T PANIC."

When I returned home I was told that my job as clinical coordinator was being eliminated. I had been given this title while I was in the hospital having my stem cell transplant. This sounded great and increased my hours and salary, but the position had been created more out of kindness and good intentions than need. Now there was a financial crunch and the clinic could not support such a position. I would need to cut back my hours. I was very anemic and the interferon increased my fatigue. Yet, I had been working hard and focusing my energy on teaching.

That night I dreamed of the burning bush. I had a vivid picture of fire burning, but not consuming the bush. Anger triggered the dream, but upon awakening, I felt energy and peace. I realized that my spirit was the bush. The energy of my anger, passion, and will, were fire and fuel for the spirit. The bush was my will to live a full and meaningful life that could not be destroyed. The dream represented my intention to persevere, to be free to use anger and not be burned by it. Chemotherapy could sear my cells but it could not consume my spirit.

Then I had a medical emergency. During a routine visit, my oncologist, Dr. Becker, noticed my fingertips were blue. To check my oxygenation she had me walk around with an oxpulse machine. It read 78. It should have been close to 100%. Immediately everyone in the clinic panicked. I was put on oxygen and rolled in a wheelchair to the nuclear medicine department to rule out a pulmonary embolism. I was also given other tests.

I had to fight not to be hospitalized and observed for the night. The next day I had a cardiogram. I did not feel sick, but I had been tired as usual. This was attributed to anemia. I also was tested in pulmonary and endocrinology. We discovered slight hypothyroidism and a drop in my heart's ejection fraction.

I had to go off the interferon that I had been taking to boost my immune system and forestall a relapse of lymphoma. I had to have my heart and thyroid function checked again. I was sent to cardiology, nuclear medicine, endocrinology, pulmonary medicine and oncology. I remember thinking that this wasn't the way I wanted to get to know the physicians at the medical center. I continued exercising and told myself repeatedly, "I will NOT panic."

It was traumatizing to have all these tests and be a patient again. Visits to doctors were taking up much of my time and it was disruptive and wearing. Each morning I would give myself Metta and continue to do so through all my tests.

Nothing serious was discovered. No one could explain what happened. Dr. Becker thought that it might have been a side effect of the interferon. Perhaps I had asthma. No one was sure, but my energy dramatically improved once I stopped the interferon. I began taking some medication for my thyroid function and my energy increased more. It was a new world! I could do much more. I had zest!

I could not bring myself to take interferon again. But going off it was a risk. As long as I was on it, I felt I was doing something to help myself stay well, yet my quality of life was diminished. No one could guarantee that interferon would increase my life span. Even if it could, I wanted to live well and have energy rather than drag around as I had been doing. I decided to go for quality, hoping it wouldn't affect longevity too much.

"Thank goodness! I feel so good now that my thyroid is regulated and I am not anemic. I cannot bear to go back on interferon and be so achy and tired again. I will take my chances. Whatever time I have to be alive I intend to experience it vividly!"

During this period, David's mother was hospitalized four times, had a pacemaker put in, still wasn't well, and had a heart attack. David's father was dying of lung cancer and we were commuting almost every other weekend to Florida. My daily meditation helped, but I still found myself struggling to maintain a state of peace. I felt as if the container that was labeled "me" was full to the brim and overflowing with wants and shoulds and wishes of what could not be.

10/19/98

Grief is arising. If only . . . If only the world, my life were perfect. Of course it isn't. Of course it can't be. While being on interferon I thought that I was doing something to prevent relapse. Now I feel a greater sense of urgency to experience each moment as perfect, special, and full. I must be wise and use every moment fully. I find myself getting upset if I am less than perfectly happy.

"Ridiculous," I tell myself. "You're just living a normal life."

Strange, now that I am better it feels harder to maintain a sense of all rightness.

In my role as senior teacher, I sat in on Jim Carmody's class. I was feeling sad, so I related to the angst I heard by class members. People were filled with doubt. How could meditation help their anxiety, their pain? They complained that they couldn't meditate; it was too unpleasant. I listened to hear how Jim responded and as I observed I was impressed not only by his words, but by the calm and caring way he steadily contained the pain being expressed, and held it so people could feel safe.

As I sat in the class and listened to the patients, it seemed that many of the patients were suffering from severe anxiety that had taken hold and firmly gripped their hearts and minds. I realized that they lacked trust and faith. Jim was showing them that underneath all the fear and pain and storms of feelings, there could be calm. This calm is equanimity.

I realize that even in the midst of my anger and self-pity, there is perspective. I do believe that my sticky, ugly feelings will pass away. They are gone now as I write this, but I know I am vulnerable and they will come again. It doesn't matter because they'll also go again.

The challenge was to maintain my faith and determination and to keep practicing — being here now — with an open heart and more accepting mind.

EXERCISE: HINDRANCES

This meditation/exercise is about allowing yourself to feel what you don't like, that which is getting in your way of peace and happiness. Name it. Write it down and then choose some art materials to creatively express the feeling or obstruction.

I'm writing this in BIG black letters because when you are in the grip of anger or doubt or fear, or whatever keeps you down we become absorbed by it and lose our ability to simply observe and be a witness. For it to pass we must bring compassion to it and get to know it better.

IF YOU LIKE YOU CAN begin this exercise by first meditating, bringing awareness to your breath and letting the mind settle and calm. Allow the name of what holds you down, or is a hindrance to your joy, to come to you. Perhaps it will be an image or a picture of a scene. Maybe it's a felt sense, a feeling or sensation. With the mind anchored to the breath and the present moment, simply observe it. Then, when you are ready, move from your meditation position to a table that you have supplied with art materials of your choice and represent this hindrance. Choose colors and forms that reflect this negativity. You can also create a collage with pictures from magazines or even fabrics. You can create an image in clay. Give yourself permission to explore and create freely. After you have done this, look at what you've created and write about it.

This can also be done as a writing exercise, but it can be very illuminating and freeing to combine the two modalities. Enjoy the process. Remember, it is a learning experience.

Everything changes. You can notice if this experience changes you and your attitude toward your challenge. Be aware of your attitude as you do this exercise. Notice when you lose interest. Notice what holds your attention. Be aware of when you feel open and when you feel closed. When you are finished, congratulate yourself for taking the time to examine something difficult. Praise yourself. You're allowed!

EXERCISE: IF ONLY. . . .

Complete this statement:

If only ——————————— then ———————————.

An example:
If only *I didn't have cancer* then *my life would be perfect.*

If only ——————————— then ———————————.

If only ——————————— then ———————————.

If only ——————————— then ———————————.

If only ——————————— then ———————————.

If only ——————————— then ———————————.

If only ——————————— then ———————————.

Now imagine what it would be like if you could let go of these "if only's." Would you be happier? Would you feel more peaceful?

STICKY FEELINGS

When the shrouds of sadness
are crushing your heart
and dampening your spirit
LOOK OUT!
Open up the window.
Smell the air.
Explore the sky.

When you feel the black clouds of grief
darkening your heart,
clouding your mind,
shrinking your world,

Breathe in and out.
Take a walk.
Play with your dog.
Have a cup of tea.

Treat your self tenderly.
It will pass.
Understanding will come
and a sweet release.

I seemed to keep learning the same lesson again and again:

Accept.
Have faith.
Trust.
Let Be.
Be compassionate and non-judgmental.

My life had returned to normal but normal wasn't what I expected. It was different from the time before I knew I had cancer. I felt older and less attractive. Chemotherapy had hastened menopause. With that came a decrease in libido and some weight gain; rather, I no longer could easily shed pounds so the weight I had gained from steroid use remained. I remember going to the wedding of a cousin's daughter. She hadn't seen me in a number of years and as I walked in she ran towards me and cried out, "Goldie."

That was my mother, not me. It blew my conception of myself as young-looking. Now, it seemed, I looked like a plump middle-aged woman. No longer did waiters flirt with me as they took my order. I was now, "Ma'am," not "Miss." I noticed I was also less adventurous and more cautious about trying new things. No longer did I plunge into the ocean, or ride the waves fearlessly. I put my toe in and stood at the line where surf met shore and hesitated, carefully plotting the best time to enter into the sea, and often, turning back to my chair.

Acceptance was the key to happiness, but the stubborn little girl in me pushed on. I didn't want *anything* to be different and of course it was. Time and again I'd say, "The more I can accept my limitations, the freer I will be."

However, it was an adjustment to know what was possible and what was too much. I feared resuming my private practice as a psychotherapist. I didn't feel I had the energy to do the intensive work it required *and* also successfully hold a class of twenty-five or more people who were in serious pain and help them feel safe. I had enjoyed balancing the two; they complemented each other.

I had to be wiser in my use of time and often had to stop to rest. As often as possible, I closed my office door, took out my yoga mat and lay down for a half-hour snooze. If I didn't, my body would be present, but fatigue would cloud my mind and decrease my enjoyment of an event, be it a get-together with friends or an evening class.

Morris died and his death triggered more sadness. I went to the funeral and wrote:

MORRIS DIED

People are talking and visiting.
It is a time of reminiscing and mourning.
Sadness resides in my throat.

My mother and father dead.
Sitting shiva gives me a migraine.

I do not feel it is proper to express my own grief.
This family corks emotion.
The bottle is not champagne.

I feel like moaning and tearing my hair . . .
loudly demonstrating grief and anger,
not at Morris's death,
But at propriety that cloaks the truth,
At the funeral parlor that made up his face so he'd look good.
At fears that make this life smaller.
And dreams never to be fulfilled

Morris was 91
I am 55.
How many days will I have with my husband to experience joy?

Can I
Accept
the way things are?

It was winter again and I felt the absence of light. I had to consciously make an effort for my sadness to lift. I sat at my desk, looked at the trees laden with snow.

The wind blows fiercely
I watch the fir branches bending
They come back upright.

To counter my sadness, it also helped to talk to friends. One day, as Christmas and Hanukkah were approaching, I called an old friend and compared strategies for feeling lighter. We talked about exercise classes and herbal remedies for cloudy mental states and heavy hearts. After we finished speaking, I drank some tea, baked some bread, and attempted a low-fat linzer torte cookie recipe using prune sauce instead of the margarine called for in the recipe. I must have used too much prune sauce because the batter became a sticky glue-like substance that stuck to my fingers and hand. I couldn't shake it off or roll it out. I wondered if this was a metaphor for my mental state. My fingers and hand were too sticky and gooey even to touch the doorknob or faucet handle to wipe off the dough. I was stuck, literally. I let the dog lick it off my hand. She loved it.

Taking a breath, I thought of the trees outside, righted myself and began again. I washed my hands, gathered another wad of dough, patted it down between plastic wrap and put it in the freezer so I could roll it out again. I wondered if I, too, needed to chill out. I couldn't put aside memories of being a cancer patient or my fear of a recurrence.

Later that day I went to the beauty parlor to have my hair cut. Cookies and chocolates were set out on the receptionist's desk, and there was a tree with gifts under it. As I helped myself to a cookie, I noticed that David, the owner, still shaved his head. It reminded me that here, two years ago, I had had my head shaved so I wouldn't have to wake with clumps of hair on my pillow.

I went to bed that night after listening to my tape of Frank Loesser's *The Most Happy Fellow*. I cried; it made me think of my mother, who had loved it. We'd be leaving in a few days to give solace to David's mom. I couldn't imagine what it would be like to be alone after 56 years of marriage. Yet, I didn't want to go to Florida. I wrote:

I'd rather have a full temper tantrum, stamp my feet and yell out, "Damn! Let's go on vacation instead. It's been a long grim time. Let's lighten up and play."

I shall have another test, a gallium scan, in a few weeks, which I dread. Not the scan itself, but the reminder that I had lymphoma. If it shows up on the scan I'll have to deal with it again. "Humbug!" Instead

I'd rather be sitting here, tapping on my keyboard, letting my mind wander. I have plans. Vacations, workshops to create. Classes to take. Challenges to meet. I do NOT want to be sidetracked. Worse yet, I do not want cancer to be my main track. No. Absolutely not!

We went to Florida, which of course was better than I had anticipated, and the time came for my gallium scan. On the morning of the scan, I opened my closet door and eyed my wardrobe. I have my clothes arranged by color: oranges, reds, bright yellow, some bright blues and black. I often dress to match my mood. Unconsciously, I chose orange, the color of Halloween, scare, and horror. It was my protest. As I entered the nuclear medicine lab, the physician commented, "You're all in orange."

While waiting for the results, I wrote:

January 25, 1999

Orange
I'm in orange today.
Orange tights, orange shirt, orange jacket.
I wore it to match my mood.
In protest I scream
Gallium Scan!
CANCER!

Disappointment.
As I re-read my journal I notice
Ups and Downs.

THIS IS IT!
"Hold it lightly.
It's all a dream."

I talk to myself.
Not liking
This,
my experience
NOW.

My brother is impressed by my equanimity.
My ability to re-focus and pay attention to what is here for me.

What can I do?
What do I have?

I wait.

Aware
of dis-ease
Not liking

Not knowing
What
the outcome will be.

More tests, more chemo?
Will I be alive to see the buds return to the trees?

Two hours later . . .

Orange is now the color of relief.
Release.
Cancer in remission.

I sit in a sushi bar in Westboro, Mass.
Mauve and Jade.
Manipulating my chopsticks.

The sun is out.
The air is crisp and cold.
My miso is warm and tasty.

Behind me two men are talking business.
In front of me are two moms with their kids.

I am again
In life
Outside of the hospital.

Life everywhere.
Here NOW.
Mortality and Impermanence forgotten as I chew
and taste my sushi.

I was happy with the test results, but grief (and anger) continued to cling to me. I went on my usual winter retreat and grief, experienced as a heaviness and tightness around the area of my heart, was predominant. My teacher, Joseph (Goldstein), described grief as a holding. This upset me. I thought he was saying that if I were good (a better meditator) I could let go, release and be happy. Then I wouldn't feel grief. I got angry; angry at being sad and angry with Joseph, thinking he was being too much of a purist, that grief was a normal part of the recovery process. I wrote a note with a little poem to him describing my grief, justifying it, and the way I worked with it.

He wrote back, "Your description of opening to the grief sounds just right. At times it might also be interesting to investigate what is underneath the grief — what thoughts or feelings condition it. This is different than fighting or resisting it — rather a gentle inquiry with much metta (love and kindness)."

This didn't satisfy me. I thought my grief was normal and natural. I decided to be compassionate toward my pain and to stop seeing it as a negative implication of my skill as a meditator. I remembered Sylvia Boorstein's words, "Sometimes it just takes awhile for pain to leave the body."

I am here on retreat to move beyond old wounds and to feel good enough, dayenu *(it's sufficient) to quiet that inner judging voice. How interesting that the same themes keep recurring. Good enough, sufficient, whole, complete. That's what I teach, acknowledging fullness and abundance, wholeness.*

I was learning how to be compassionate and patient with myself. I realized that as long as I am here, alive, there will always be something that's sticky. My goal was to reach a place of balance that was roomy enough to hold my joy *and* sadness, and to have my regrets and longings float, like the clouds moving through the sky.

MEDITATION: GETTING UNSTUCK

There are times to meditate and times to act. Sometimes it is necessary to act rather than to sit. The more resources we have available to work with negative feelings the easier it is to return to a state of balance. For this exercise think about resources and actions available to help you move from a stuck position to one of greater freedom.

FIRST GET INTO YOUR meditation position and ground yourself by bringing attention to your breath. You may choose any of the meditations in this book, or simply STOP and let your mind focus on what helps you feel empowered and positive. It can be a person or group of people, it can be an activity, and it can be a thought or a particular memory. Perhaps a show tune will pop into awareness, or a memory of a teacher or a particular time that makes you smile.

Write it down. You can add to this list as ideas come to you. Take it out when you need a reminder that there are ways you can get unstuck and feel better. Your attitude is VERY important, but it helps to have a list of aids handy to use when your spirit flags.

If you are feeling particularly stuck, spend a longer time in meditation. You may need to consciously bring forth a sense of sanctuary, imagining yourself in an abode that is restful and serene. You can open your eyes and describe it in words or pictures.

Rehearse this scene in your mind until you feel confident (or almost sure) that you can reach this place.

When you are firmly there, imagine yourself unstuck. What would that look like, feel like? What would you be doing?

When you have a clear picture and feel it bodily, note it. Practice makes perfect. Treat your limitations tenderly and you will be surprised what transpires. Even stickiness passes.

Remember, you have choices. Every next moment is a new and precious moment. Explore and experiment; you can even use black humor. Be creative and trust yourself and your desire for health.

After awhile, meditation will become a sanctuary. Your ability to create space around grief and pain, and breathe into it, will expand and it will not be problematic.

SECTION IV

Tuning In And Moving Out

For years, I had been tuning into my body, beginning at my toes and working my way up to my head. The body never lied; if I was stressed, I'd feel tightness. It was often located in my neck and shoulders or sometimes my belly. Every now and then, I'd tune into my position as I sat in my chair, listening to patients. If I was working too hard or straining to make something happen, I'd find myself leaning forward with my shoulders by my ears and my chin thrust forward, my neck stiff. This told me to back off, relax, and stop pushing to make something happen. I'd take a deeper breath and physically move back into my chair and wait for my breath to slow.

I also tuned into thoughts and feelings (especially to what I didn't like), in the hope of using that information to make better choices. When I meditated, I was discovering that my fatigue, though lessened by being off interferon, still had not disappeared. To continue living fully and being effective in my work, I had to make changes. I couldn't do everything I wanted to do all at once; it needed to be incremental. I began to accept my restless, striving nature. My health stabilized, but ever present was the thought that this, too, was temporary. I wanted to squeeze in as much as I could, while I could.

I started thinking about leaving the University of Massachusetts and returning to private practice and being a consultant again. This would give me more flexibility and I could create new programs based on the mindfulness model. Yet, the thought of leaving my home, my family at The Center of Mindfulness, saddened me. It had been so much of my life for so many years, sustaining me through my single days in Cambridge, my marriage, the death of my father and now cancer. The Clinic and I had grown up together. Yet, Jon, the founder, had left the hospital, though he stayed connected to our program. Ferris, my buddy and co-teacher, had turned sixty and also left. The hospital was also changing. It had merged with another hospital in Worcester and, due to a financial crisis, had booted out our clinic. For six months, we didn't know whether we'd survive. While Saki, who was now the director of the Center, negotiated with the medical school to house us as it had done before the hospitals merged, staff had to be cut and the number of classes reduced. Morale dipped down.

My teaching continued as a bright spot. I was doing new work on the transplant unit, which engrossed me. To my great surprise, I discovered that I had become an icon of courage and determination. A picture of me and my dog, Chaya, and the text of a newspaper article (see illustration on previous page) hung in the blood donor room to inspire people to give blood. The staff on the transplant unit had been impressed by my ability to use my breathing to calm myself and cope with the stresses of mouth sores, pneumonia, and low blood counts. It seemed that no one had been able to last solely on oxygen without going on a respirator, as long as I had — a testament to meditation and an accomplishment I would not care to repeat or boast about.

Pam Doyle, a nurse practitioner on the transplant unit who was interested in applying meditation to transplant patients, took our internship program and suggested we do a small research project on meditation's effectiveness to reduce suffering. She asked if I'd be interested in bringing meditation to the unit. We met with Jon, who thought this was a great idea, and Dr. Karen Ballen, who headed the unit. Though we had no grant money, we decided to try it. This was a wonderful opportunity to give back to others some of what I had so generously received.

When I open the sealed door of the transplant unit for the first time since I had left, I felt as if I was walking into a fire . . . my own. Memories of what it was like when I was the patient returned to me. As I walked down the hallway to the nurse's station, unassisted and without tubes or an IV pole, gratitude filled me. I remembered my vulnerability and the intense discomfort of mouth sores, nausea, and general physical weakness. I also remembered those who sat with me and had been uplifting. I hoped that I could now convey some of the same peace.

The transplant unit was small. I felt joyous to be able to walk in and out of it freely. The study was experimental, so I had no set agenda. We had written up a protocol, but it was loose enough to give me the freedom simply to listen to patients and individualize the meditation instructions in words that would be meaningful to them.

My first patient was a woman who was very afraid and worried about her son who was now home alone. He had a drinking problem. As she calmed and quieted, tears came. She began talking about her fears and hurt. She didn't think her son would visit her; she felt alone and scared. I listened and then had her gently move her attention back to her breath. Speaking in a soothing voice, I suggested that she release these worrisome thoughts on the exhalation and, on the inhalation, let herself settle more deeply into the bed. I recommended that she feel the bed supporting her and feel the covers around her and focus on the sounds in the room and my voice.

I meditated with this patient three times one week and twice the next and subsequent weeks. She reported she was practicing and had used her breath awareness when her catheter was taken out and replaced by a new one. She still worried, but felt comforted and more at ease in the hospital. Slowly, her mind quieted as she learned to redirect her attention to the here and now, one breath at a time, inhalation and exhalation. Slowly, she realized that it wasn't productive to worry excessively; that her work was to survive and care for herself so she could recover and have the strength to deal with her problems later.

We also called in a psych consult to talk to her further about her family situation. This woman was not psychologically oriented, nor would she have ever sought meditation on her own. It was impressive that she had learned to incorporate it into her day, using it when she got anxious or needed to sleep. She found it soothing.

When a patient elected to be in the study, I'd go over to the unit, explain meditation to them, and sit with them. Frequently, people wanted to isolate themselves when they felt sick or nauseous. I explained that that was often a time when it was most helpful to have a person present, someone who could sit with them and simply send them good wishes (a Metta meditation). There was no need to feel ashamed. Sometimes I gave permission to feel rotten and complain. Some people thought they were being bad or weak if they were having negative thoughts. It was a relief for them to know that this was normal.

I encouraged people to breathe in relaxation and peace and breathe out toxins, or "anything that doesn't help you heal." We would breathe together, my breath matching theirs, tuning into the rhythm of life in the room — breath, sounds, sensations, thoughts, and feelings. By simply observing the flow, we witnessed impermanence; no two moments were exactly alike. Sometimes a sense of a larger presence would enter, an experience of connection not only to family and friends or others in the hospital, patients and staff, but a force greater than ourselves, of God or nature, depending on a person's belief system. There was room for awe.

Together, we sat and listened and observed, practicing, allowing whatever entered the stream of awareness. We also practiced sight meditation, looking at mementos from home, or inspirational cards, or photos of friends and family that were posted on the bulletin board in the patient's room. I listened to descriptions of loved ones. In this preliminary study, there was no specific agenda other than being mindful and present to the moment as it unfolded. Whatever arose in conversation was fine.

One day when I was sitting with a patient, I got caught in fear. The patient's skin was red, flushed by fever. She was very uncomfortable and breathing coarsely. It was clear she was scared. Outside, it was raining. I felt a tightening in my chest, a lump in my throat, the increased pounding in my heart. And then my gaze turned to the window, opaque with moisture. Droplets of water dotted the expanse of glass. I watched as the drops slowly and gently descended. I began quieting. I listened to the sound of the rain and calmed some more. My heartbeat slowed. I could guide the patient to shift her focus and watch the drops of moisture, as they gently rolled down the window in a rhythm, slow and steady. It was absorbing. We were both here, now in this moment, at peace.

Pam Doyle left the medical center for another position. The study continued with my good friend and colleague, Dr. Susan Bauer-Wu, as a principal investigator, now heading the Phyllis Cantor Institute at the Dana Farber Cancer Institute. We have extended this work to that institution. A feasibility study has been completed and published, and a more comprehensive study is being planned in conjunction with other hospitals.

Time passed without any major medical event. My goals and mottos did not change. In the year, 2000, on retreat, I kept no notes, but continued to walk and sit and tend the hurts of my heart and watch my mind observe the passage of time and change. I celebrated the twentieth anniversary of the Stress Reduction Clinic. The party to honor Jon, and his founding of the clinic, was in the backyard of our house under a huge tent. We had a live band and wonderful food. Friends and members of the stress reduction family were all gathered together in celebration. I marveled that I'd been a part of this community for all but three of its years. The work had been fulfilling and meaningful and the time had swiftly passed.

The study on the transplant unit came to an end and summer rolled around again. Once again, we went to the beach. This time Bekka didn't visit, but her parents joined us for a few days. Each morning after my meditation, David and I would stop at the bakery on the way to the beach, eat a sugar donut (giving a small piece to Chaya), park the car at the small parking lot by the beach, and go for our walk. It was a daily ritual. David was grayer, with a little less hair, but he still walked faster than I did and was skinnier.

Chaya ran ahead of us as we lathered up with suntan lotion in the parking lot. We walked down the path to the beach, stopped where the path met sand, took off our sandals and lined them up with the other shoes shed by other dog owners. We moved on, climbing up a small incline to a ridge that overlooked the beach and a view of the nearby salt pond. At this point, David and I always paused and took in the view of sea and sky. We'd note the weather of the day and listen for the sound of birds. I'd notice the light and the complement of sky, sea and sand, and their colors of browns, blues and blue-grays, interspersed with greens of beach grass and reds from the iron rich soil. The perspective of bay, beach, sea, and sand never ceased to inspire us.

Hand-in-hand, David and I walked down to the shore, Chaya in the lead, running ahead to take her morning dip. We'd wait for her and then she'd run along with us, sometimes stopping to nuzzle or be sniffed by another dog, as we walked along the crescent-shaped beach to a large boulder about a mile down the shore. Sometimes we'd stop to chat with another dog owner. We walked carefully, stepping around the many small stones the waves had deposited on the beach.

Each morning, the light would be different, the tide at a different spot, and we'd spy new stones half-buried in the sand or glittering in the light. We made a game of spotting "perfect" white ones to carry home for the rock garden in our living room. We examined each stone carefully. They needed to be smooth and have a shape, pattern, or color that pleased us. A few we pocketed as treasures to carry home; the others we threw back into the sand.

As I walked, eyeing the stones, I reflected on the action of the waves that deposited them on the shore, carving and shaping them with the help of wind and weather, sea and air, to give them their distinctive character. I couldn't help but compare them to our lives. Together, they formed the ground on which we walked.

The large boulder that was our destination had a large crack in it. Each year, we had noticed the crack's deepening, as it began to cleave the rock in two. One week, we saw an artist perched beside it with his sketchpad and watercolors. At the end of the summer, we found his picture hanging in a gallery. It captured a moment of light and tide and rock, a moment in time that no longer exists.

As I write, the stones we chose to bring home rest in my living room by my plants and a small fountain. I have placed a laughing

Buddha nearby. It is a reminder of sun and sand, days of leisure and the beauty to be found in the wear and tear of life. It also reminds me of impermanence.

During the summer of 2001 we went to the beach in July, not in August as is our custom. That August, three stress reduction teachers — Melissa, Ferris, and I — went to Wales to run a teacher-training program for the mindfulness teachers in the program that Mark Williams had created at the University of Bangor. He, John Teasdale, and Zindl Siegal, who had worked with us on their mindfulness-based cognitive therapy program for depression, were present, along with some other European teachers. Jon and Saki led a conference first and we followed them. Our training was in-depth and intimate, with perhaps twenty-five teachers, primarily those who worked with Mark. I was excited. Melissa and I traveled a bit first, stopping in Bath. I visited Stonehenge. Then we went to the retreat center. It was the first time I had traveled abroad to do a training session and I thought that if I were to leave the clinic, the trip to Wales would be a wonderful way to end my teaching years at the Center.

Throughout the training, as our minds quieted, mine thought, should I or should I not leave the clinic? Was it time for me to go? Melissa and Florence, who I had brought on, were now mature teachers. Jon had left, Ferris had left, and I'd be turning sixty in another couple of years. I still fatigued easily. Was it time for a change? By the end of the retreat I thought, "Yes, I can do this." I planned to stay connected, but I was ready for a fresh relationship with the Center and my work. I decided to give notice. When I returned.

I walked into Saki's office to resign. It was Tuesday morning, September 11, 2001.

MEDITATION: TRUSTING THE PROCESS: LETTING THE PATH UNFOLD

Listening to what is true and having it inform our actions is a process requiring trust, time, and commitment. It may also mean taking chances and making some changes in the way we are living our lives. Change is always a stressor but is inevitable. It may be necessary if we want to renew ourselves and be free.

LET YOUR MIND QUIET and be still, like that still forest pool. To do this, you may choose any of the meditations that resonate with you. It is important to give yourself sufficient time to be like that reflecting pool and let things come and go. Thoughts, sensations, sounds, and feelings can be like ripples on the pond. Your awareness can reside deep down under the surface where there is calm. Do your best to open to whatever appears, be they wonders or not, but keep your attention in this moment.

When you feel that your attention is steady and the mind has quieted, you can use this time to reflect on the events of the day. Let your mind review the activities of your day. What engaged you? What did not? What did you do out of obligation? What did you do out of choice? Did that affect how you perceived the event?

Notice the people that you came into contact with during the day. What was the nature of the relationship and the interaction between you? Was there a feeling of satisfaction, boredom, restlessness, aversion, or receptivity? What type of communication was it? What was the intention behind it? Did it fulfill its purpose? How satisfying was it?

What choices did you make today? Were you aware of the choices as they occurred? Were they acceptable to you? If you could redo your day, would you do anything different? Simply notice, without judging, as you do this review.

You may want to do this for more than one day, focusing on one particular aspect of the day. Notice what brings aversion (a pushing away), or clinging (you want to hold on). All are fine. You may ask yourself: Am I acting ethically?

How fulfilling and honest is this action or event? Is this in harmony with my goals? Does it have a purpose? Does it give me meaning? Is it important for the well-being of others and myself? Does it contribute to a fulfilling life?

It is useful to do this assessment more than once, and at different times of day and on different days. Use it simply to gather information. DO NOTHING but SIMPLY OBSERVE. Regularly practicing mindfulness and trusting the process can guide you to deeper levels of meaning and authenticity. If your commitment is to living fully and wholly, your observations will help you make choices that will be correct. Treat yourself kindly and tenderly, trusting your own inner wisdom to do this. All you have to do is to listen and follow what you know to be true.

9/11 AND NEW VENTURES

That Tuesday morning, when I listened to the radio on my way to the Center, I heard that some smoke had been coming out of the World Trade Towers, but I had no idea of the catastrophe that was to unfold. My mind was filled with the enormity of my decision to resign. As I was talking to Saki and explaining my reasons for taking this BIG step of venturing out on my own, Jeanie Baril, our administrative assistant, banged on the door and rushed in.

"A plane flew into the trade tower!" she exclaimed.

"No!"

"Yes."

Stunned, we listened to the news in horror, my own news now eclipsed by this tragedy. The date, the time, became seared into memory. I realized that life would be different from now on, for us all.

A few days later, when I went to Hope Lodge, where Susan Bauer-Wu and I led a support group for cancer patients that revolved around meditation and creative therapies, art and writing, followed by head and neck massages, we discovered that the patients weren't as surprised or shocked by 9/11 as others. Their diagnosis of cancer had been their personal equivalent of 9/11 and the explosion that shook the world. Living with a life-threatening disease had already upset their sense of order and undermined their feelings of inviolability. They were living with the knowledge that they could be attacked by cancer at any time. Before 9/11 their worlds had already changed, never to be the same.

I understood perfectly. I was a facilitator for the group, but I had begun it in part to help me understand and move through my own vulnerability. By helping others cope with their loss and fear of death, I was helping myself cope with my own sadness and loss of innocence. We will all die, but none of us know how and when, myself included, and I couldn't forget that. I did know I preferred it to be later; not now. I did know I wanted to live as fully and wisely as possible, for as long as I could.

Aachan Chah, a meditation master wrote:

Try to be mindful and let things take their natural course.
Then your mind will become clear in any surroundings,
like a clear forest pool.
All kinds of wonderful rare animals will come to drink in the pool,
and you will see clearly the nature of all things.
You will see many strange and wonderful things come and go,
but you will be still.
This is the happiness of mindfulness.

I was happy. I loved working in the Stress Reduction Clinic, now called the Center for Mindfulness, but it was time for a change. I needed to experiment, and let my bubbly, spontaneous, wild, irreverent, wise self be adventurous. I helped the stress reduction program reach maturity and in so doing, I also grew up. I felt like a teenager leaving the family and going out on her own. I was curious to see what forms MBSR would take in my life and how I would adapt it to work with cancer patients and in settings other than the medical school. I also wanted more time to write and explore my own creativity.

"You are your own best teacher," I tell people.

Now, whether I sit with a cancer patient or I am working as a psychotherapist, my goal continues to help others access their own wisdom and strength.

I teach a meditation class at Dana Farber Cancer Institute through the Zakim Center's integrative medicine program. This class is open to staff, patients, and family members. In one session people learn to focus on a neutral object, like sound or the breath, which is occurring in the present moment. Sometimes, after following our breath in an upright position, we do a bodyscan.

One day, one of the participants did not want to miss the class, but had no daycare for her five-year-old son. She brought him with her. As I spoke, and his mother meditated, he snuggled into her lap. When we finished and transitioned into the bodyscan and Mom moved to lie supine on the floor, he also changed his position to accommodate to her. He stretched out and rested his head on her belly. As she breathed, so did he. Normally he was a very active boy but now he was quiet and gave his mother some time to rest. We all were enchanted and settled into the meditation, smiling.

Sometimes in this drop-in class we do Metta. The sessions are brief, but often potent. One young man, who came with itching he described as excruciating, learned to breathe with the sensations, and after one session, with practice at home, found relief.

As people learn more about my work, they sometimes call me for advice. One morning, as I was working on this book, the phone rang. It was a woman who had seen my name in the newspaper. She knew I was a cancer patient and was doing something for cancer patients involving meditation. She was going to have surgery for ovarian cancer the next day. She told me that she was fasting in preparation for her surgery. She was scared and needed some affirmation that she could get through this.

"I've been feeling good," she told me. "Discovering I have cancer is a shock. I feel like this news is a death sentence. I was just diagnosed last week."

I listened to her and recommended some funny videos to watch to take her mind off the next day's surgery. I don't think it mattered what I said. She needed to talk, preferably to someone else who had cancer and was alive and well. I'm glad she had the courage to reach out and I had the luck to be present.

As I write this, I'm planning other programs and talks, including the interface of meditation and psychotherapy. I've resumed my private practice as a psychotherapist, as well as some group work incorporating meditation with art and writing. I'm also teaching first year medical students at the University of Massachusetts Medical School and continue to participate in the Center for Mindfulness and its conference and professional training program. I've also been fortunate enough to lead week-long programs at Rancho La Puerta, a wonderful spa, in *Awakening the Spirit* with Phyllis Pilgrim, *Facing Challenge with Grace*, and *Mindful Living*.

I'm challenged to keep creating and trust what unfolds. I feel blessed. Just yesterday I taught meditation at an assisted living center. Who knows, perhaps I, too, shall grow old.

FOR NOW

Dropping down
Lower and lower.
The quiet grows within.

Doing nothing
My wanting mind stills.

In the silence
In the space

What
I have been seeking
Is found.

It is nothing
Less than everything
and
More than anything.

Being here
For now
Now.

When struggle ceases and stillness comes,
it is easy to be mindful and let things take their natural course.

❧

MEDITATION: COMMITTING TO PRACTICE

Change is never easy. It was hard for me to change my relationship to the clinic that was such a large part of my life. To do so I needed to listen and trust my own inner wisdom and voice. I needed to trust that my dear friends and the work I so loved could continue as a part of me. In opening to my truth I found myself becoming more alive. I was learning to trust that through deep listening, consistent practice and intention, right action springs forth.

By now, if you've read this book through, you've been exposed to different meditations: the sitting meditation with awareness of breathing, a bodyscan meditation and Metta, loving-kindness meditations.

Choose one of these meditations and make a commitment to practice it daily. Choose the length of time for your practice. Write it down or make a mental note of when you will practice. Choose your environment carefully and let it be your spot, an oasis of tranquility and peace that you can return to for practice. You can treat yourself to a timer so you won't have to look at a clock or worry about the time.

Begin the meditation of your choice and allow insights to arise without any expectation as to what might happen. If there is a question you have or something you need to know, you can form it in your mind before you meditate, but then let it go. The answer will come to you if you give it time and space and continue your commitment to practice. The more you let yourself simply observe what happens and bring your attention to your direct experience, moment by moment, the greater will be your ability to discover what you need in order to care for yourself wisely. The attitude that you bring to this practice will fuel the process. It is important and needs to travel with you on the meditation cushion and off.

You can extend your practice throughout the day in an informal way. Choose activities that you do habitually, such as brushing your teeth and washing your hands, waiting in line, or driving your car. For example, when you are at a stoplight, STOP. Bring your attention into your body. Be aware of your breathing, feel the breath and notice the position of your body. Are your hands gripping the wheel? Are you leaning forward or back? You can use this time to return to the present moment, breathing consciously with it, listening to sounds, breathing in the scents around you and experiencing physical sensations. The more often you stop, returning home to the present moment, the easier it will be to tame the monkey of a mind we all have. Then, insight can enter and with it wisdom and freedom from suffering.

There will always be wear and tear if you are dedicated to living a full life, but it is possible to have equanimity and stay fresh and awake — if you make a decision to do so. Crisis can wake us up, but how wonderful it is to develop our practice when conditions are calm. Let the wear and tear of life highlight beauty within and without. Experience and time can smooth out rough edges and create treasures to be held and loved for all time. Be patient and trust, and maintain a regular practice. Happiness is possible as long as you can be open to your experience, whatever it may be.

Practice. Practice. Practice. Now!

WRITE DOWN WHEN YOU WILL PRACTICE.

WRITE DOWN WHERE YOU WILL PRACTICE.

INCLUDE INFORMAL PRACTICE.
I will tune into my body when. . . . (e.g. the phone rings). *I will bring awareness to my breath when.* . . . (I'm waiting in line at the store.)

Surrender To What Is

In anticipation of my sixtieth birthday, I gave myself the present of a loving-kindness meditation retreat with two of my favorite teachers, Kamala Masters and Sharon Salzberg. It was a beautiful spring day and I was finishing my walk around the loop, a two-and-a-half-mile road by the Insight Meditation Society in Barre, Massachusetts where I was meditating. As I walked, I repeated rhythmically to myself the phrases of the loving-kindness meditation, "May I be safe and protected. May I be happy and peaceful. May I be healthy and strong. May I live with ease."

Sometimes I'd forget "healthy and strong." My mind would note this and then, more fervently, I'd repeat to myself, "May I be healthy and strong," and continue on.

I was feeling healthy and strong. It felt good to be moving my body briskly after the long hours of sitting still in the Meditation Hall or slowly walking and concentrating on the phrases of the meditation. It was dusk, the black flies seemed to have retired for the night, and the green freshness of spring filled my nostrils as I planted my feet on the ground. I felt strong and protected, peaceful, happy and at ease when I felt a sharp pain in my lower right side.

I continued on, but the pain didn't abate and it became painful to move. It was surprising, but I continued simply to notice and breathe with it and returned to the hall, concerned I'd be late for the night's Dharma talk. I couldn't be having appendicitis, could I?

During the talk, my concentration was fully focused on Kamala as she described a time when her meditation teacher, Munindra-ji, had visited her and she was trying to appear to be a "good meditator" with a perfect family life. Of course, she, and we, knew that this desire for perfection could only be a setup for disappointment and suffering. Nothing is quite as we want it to be, even "perfect families." That night, Kamala's youngest daughter Terese, then 10, and her daughter's father got into a shouting match which culminated in Terese leaving the table and slamming the door to her room.

"Open that door!" yelled Terese's dad.

"No!" screamed Terese.

"Open it or I'll knock it down."

"Go ahead!"

Mortified, Kamala listened, powerless to intercede. She put her head down on the table. With great compassion, Munindra-ji softly tapped her on the arm and said, "Surrender to the law." (The natural moment-to-moment unfolding of how things are.)

Kamala went on to describe how helpful it has been to remember her teacher's compassion and the wisdom of his words when she finds herself in difficult and unpleasant circumstances.

"Accept what is true. Surrender to what is true."

My pain subsided as I sat, but afterward it still hurt to get up and walk. I didn't like this. I found it hard to believe that my body was in distress. Memories of Kamala, sitting in my room in the hospital sending me Metta when I was sick with pneumonia and on a respirator following my stem cell transplant, returned to me.

This couldn't be serious, could it? I thought.

Remembering Kamala's story, I noted my resistance.

How could this be happening?

I made a conscious effort not to resist what I was feeling. I didn't panic. I watched the pain and my disbelieving mind. I hoped the sharp sensations on the right side of my abdomen would just disappear. Continuing to observe the changing sensations and repeat Metta to myself, I went to bed, only to wake up a few hours later in severe pain. It was difficult to move, but with Metta I went back to sleep.

In the morning, concerned, I unearthed my cell phone, which we weren't supposed to use while on retreat or in the building (the walls were too thin and it was disruptive). I gathered my jacket and went outside into the early morning mist to call David.

"Is the pain below your belly button?" he asked.

"Yes."

"Call your primary care physician," he said.

I ate breakfast, but the pain continued. I called my doctor.

"Am I having an appendicitis?" I asked.

"I can't feel your belly over the phone," she responded wisely. "Go to the health center near you. I'll approve it."

In-breath, out-breath.

May I be safe and protected.
May I be happy and peaceful.
May I be healthy and strong.
May I live with ease.

The pain intensified. Now worried that I might be having a ruptured appendix, I called the health center and got an appointment for later in the afternoon.

I went to my group interview with Sharon Salzberg.

"How's it going?" she asked.

Sharon had sent me a card when I had my stem cell transplant. I was calm, my mind was quiet. I did not want to acknowledge I might be having another medical emergency.

"I'm having some pain," I said. "If it continues, I'll deal with it."

Sharon skillfully answered questions and I remember talking about equanimity.

The pain worsened. I couldn't bend over to tie my shoelaces.

May I be safe and protected.
Surrender to what is true.

At the medical clinic, they weren't sure what was happening. They thought I might be having an early appendicitis and told me to observe it longer. I called David again and he told me to come home immediately.

"I'll come home *after* the Dharma talk," I told him. Home is only forty minutes away and I still didn't want to admit something was really wrong with me. This interrupted my plan for the week.

May I be safe and protected.
May I be happy.
May I be healthy and strong.
May I live with ease.

I told the staff at IMS I'd be leaving, but I hoped to return. Should I empty my room, or was it possible this pain was fleeting and I could return to the retreat?

Surrender to what is true.

I compromised and packed my clothes, but left my sheets on the bed and my shawl over my seat in the meditation hall . . . just in case.

In the office, as I said good-bye, one of the staff looked at me. I was calm, quiet, standing upright, and not in apparent agony.

"Do you have any thoughts as to why this is happening on retreat?" he asked inquisitively.

"Many thoughts," I said, "None of which I am going to think about . . . things happen."

"I've had lymphoma," I said. "Everyone panics, but I must attend to this."

He looked at me. "Yes," he said. "Things happen."

Later that night, as I lay on a stretcher in the emergency room, I repeated the Metta Meditation to myself. I continued doing so as I drank the contrast for a CAT scan, as I waited through the night and the next day to clear out my bowels, as I prepared for surgery, and as I awoke from surgery. I felt bathed in love and light. The words comforted me and rang true.

May I be safe and protected.
May I be happy.
May I be healthy.
May I live with ease.

I survived surgery. I didn't have an abscess or appendicitis, but the lymphoma was back, this time in the form of a small tumor, about nine centimeters, attached to my colon. Fortunately, the surgeon was able to remove it and I didn't need an ostomy. The pain had been caused by the cessation of blood flow to the tumor. How interesting that this had happened while I was on retreat. Some wondered if the Metta I had practiced had affected the cessation of blood to the tumor. The oncologist doubted it, but who knows? No other spots appeared on my CAT scans or in my belly. Yet, I was back in the cycle of tests and doctors and office visits. One oncologist recommended I have a bone marrow transplant. Another said, "Let's wait and watch."

The future . . . who knows? I do know that I feel safe and protected, happy, healthy, and able to live with ease . . . and with cancer. How blessed I am to be here, now. How blessed I am to have friends and loved ones. How blessed I am to feel blessed. May we all live with ease and be happy. May we all be healthy. May we all be safe and protected.

What a relief to accept what is true and not resist in vain.

My work continues. I celebrated my sixtieth birthday in June with my stem cell sisters. Agnetha, who is Swedish, surprised me and made a cake and wove a daisy chain for me to wear. Summer came and went. Bekka visited us on the Vineyard; she is now eighteen and has finished her first year of college. Her boyfriend came for a day and David and I went kayaking with them. They were impressed that we could keep up. So were we. We still walked along the beach with Chaya and pocketed a few stones. I ate my morning sugar donut without feeling guilty. I gazed at the sea and sky and thought:

May we all be well . . . and Here . . . for Now . . . Now.

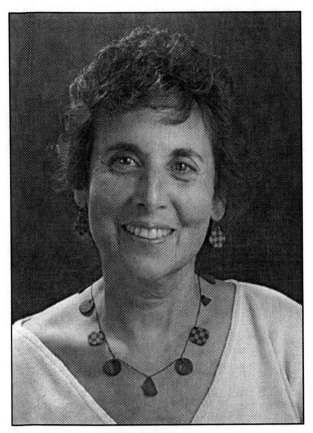

Elana Rosenbaum, MS, LICSW, integrates her years of experience as a psychotherapist with her practice of insight meditation to help people live fully and well, whether they are cancer patients or coping with the stress of daily life. She is adjunct faculty at the Center for Mindfulness in Medicine, Healthcare and Society, where, for over eighteen years, she was a senior instructor in mindfulness-based stress reduction. She has taught meditation to cancer patients on the transplant unit in hospitals and outpatient settings, including the Dana Farber Cancer Institute. She also teaches at the University of Massachusetts Medical School. She is founder of Mindful Living (www.mindfuliving.com) and co-founder of Retreats to Renew, providing training and workshops for spas, businesses, healthcare organizations, and educational institutions.

Elana lives in Worcester, Massachusetts with her husband David and Springer spaniel, Chaya (Life).

Printed in the United States
92649LV00002B/159/A